QUESTIONS
from those who
KNOW

CINDY JUSINO & JEANETTE BAKER

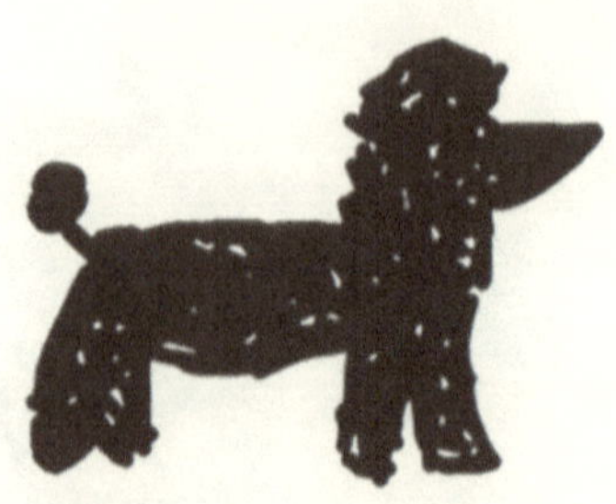

First American Paperback
Book One
Cover Design by Christina Fuselli

Sensational Publications
P.O. Box 445
Geneva IL 60134
www.SensationalPublications.com

Paperback ISBN: 978-0-9912808-1-0
EBook ISBN: 978-0-9912808-4-1
Library of Congress Control Number: 2013921988

Contents

Introduction 1

Cindy Jusino...5

Jeanette Baker 9

Erica Cornell 13

Morgan L Masterson 15

Shannon Bussells 17

Kristen S. 20

Christie Spence 23

Angela Slate..26

Marzena Walker 28

Sharon Walsh 33

Karly Montsion 36

Sherry Johnstone 40

Ronetta Fosnaugh 42

Lila Lins 44

Jax..47

Dana 50

Sarah Chagnot..52

Charity Ponton 54

Rachel Pigue 57

Kristie Clocksin 61

Laura Smith 64

Mary Camp..67

BTE Mom...69

Lora Sweeney 71

Sonya...74

KJB 76

Jamie Murray 78

Amy Bakken 80

Patricia 83

Danyell Pemerton 85

Candice Nichols 89

Momma with SPD child 94

Sally Hoyt 96

Kirstie Steptoe 99

Ingrid Fehr 101

Naomi Mae Conto 105

Alexandria Glare 107

Jillian Hill 110

Kelli Flores 113

Sandy M Palmer 116

Dorinda Richardson 118

Sarah Heard 121

Shandi M. Foster 123

Mary Kemper 127

Rachel 131

Cassandra I. Coleman 133

Dr. Amanda M. Vaden 137

Julie Foser 140

Jo Miller 145

Jennifer S. 148

Angie Carlozzi 152

Pam Root 156

Rebecca Waldron 159

Karen Ogden 163

Sydney Platt 166

Hayley Kairewich 169

Poems..174

Links and More:..180

Introduction

This book is my attempt at helping fellow parents and caregivers of children with Sensory Processing Disorder. When my own son was diagnosed at the age of two, I spent countless hours researching and trying to find the best ways to help him.

On the web you can find a mix of ideas that can be overwhelming at times. I decided that what we really needed was some tried and true advice from the real experts, from the parents and caregivers that are living though this. In these pages you will find real people implementing strategies and giving advice on caring for a child with Sensory Processing Disorder. I hope that what you read helps you on your journey, at the very least I hope it brings encouragement to know that you are not alone.

The one thing I do want to point out is that I really do believe it gets better. It may not be noticed from one day to the next, but I find that when I look back at how things were a year or two ago I can really see how we have progressed over time.

-Cindy M. Jusino

This book contains real stories from real parents who are all too familiar with Sensory Processing Disorder. This book will comfort you in times of questioning, frustration and confusion. Some stories you will be able to relate to more than others as all children with Sensory Processing Disorder are different and have different needs and behaviors.

I have never been sure about what I have wanted to do with my life other than be a mom, help others and be a writer. I started researching special needs in 2007 when Bean had been given her Sensory Processing Disorder diagnosis. I wanted to learn as much as I could to help her and improve our family situation. The more I began to read and learn, the more I wanted a place to go with others who could understand what I was going through.

I couldn't find many resources so I decided to start a website and build my own Facebook pages. I wanted to build a community - an SPD family that would be made up of people from all over the world. Every day I would look and see the "likes" getting higher and higher, and before I knew it I was over 15,000. I wanted to continue to find different ways to help Bean, others and myself. I spoke to Cindy Jusino about writing books and the idea for this book was born and seemed absolutely brilliant to me.

I remember back to when I wanted to know about Sensory Processing Disorder. I had so many questions. What doctors do I need to take Bean to? What therapies will she need? Will this go away? What items to buy, what caused this and am I the only one experiencing this? This book will give a very clear picture of what to expect, how to get a diagnosis and most importantly will reassure you that you are not alone. There are many others who experience this every day all around the world. It's not just you.

Being a mom of one child at 17 was difficult. Having a child so young I definitely did not prepare myself for what was to come and how my life would be about to change. I thought being a mom would be fun, amazing and so fulfilling. Yes, it was and has been, but even the smallest tasks were all difficult from bathing, eating and even sleeping. Tantrums all day long. Wow, the tantrums were the toughest part of my day. After four more years I found out I was having another child. I was already not able to leave the house because of the behaviors. I knew the chances of this happening again were possible. Filled with fear of the unknown, I didn't imagine in a million years I was about to have another child with many more diagnoses than the first child.

I started to notice after I had my second child she was very different but in many ways the same as the first one. She wanted to be naked, couldn't wear any clothes, she didn't want to sleep and when she did it was very little. She would get very over stimulated by the smallest things and it would result in meltdowns. She was always overheated, wearing flip flops and shorts in minus fifty weather. She was constantly seeking messy play, couldn't have bed sheets or blankets on her bed, hugs needed to be at her request and she wiped off her kisses, couldn't socialize like other children, she was always in constant motion, couldn't seem to sit still at all, she was always climbing, bouncing, jumping and spinning. Now I understand why, she is a seeker! I didn't know what a seeker was back then but I sure do now.

After a while of running Facebook groups and pages my situation, the diagnosis, the research, what other parents had to say, it all began to fit together like a puzzle. I now understand why she doesn't like clothes but most importantly I learned about brushing and joint compressions to help her. I now know why every time sirens go off while we are out she has to cover her ears and how to help her. Learning about Sensory Processing Disorder can be a lot of information to learn and understand. We could read every day for the rest of our lives about it and still never learn it all. I want this book to be a way to give others that understanding. To be able to listen to the stories from other parents who live with these experiences without all the big words that nobody understands.

The Sensory Processing Disorder community would be the best place to begin. Who better to ask than those parents who have children who have been diagnosed with SPD and live the experience every day. As I researched I realized I also have SPD, I have finally been given the opportunity to not just understand Bean but myself too, as through several years I wasn't able to understand this and believed I was just different.

I want others to read this book so they too can see understand why we are different and feel the ways we do and understand our children better. I have been inspired by many stories and it is my honor to be able to share some of these stories with you. Grab a blanket, sit back, get comfortable and get ready to not only understand Sensory Processing Disorder but to also feel a place of belonging.

-Jeanette Baker

Cindy Jusino

St. Charles, IL

1. When did you first notice your child had Sensory Processing Disorder? When and how was he/she officially diagnosed?

I noticed since birth that there was something different about my now 4 year old son. He couldn't stand riding in the car and would cry from the second I put him in until the second I got him out. He would also need constant stimulation, I could never just leave him to sit on the floor for a few minutes to play. He had to constantly be bounced around the house. He was officially diagnosed by a team at a local hospital at two and a half, although his Occupational Therapist and our mother in-law (who works with special needs children) had already told us he had it. With our second son, who is now 1, we called Early Interventions for speech therapy and were shocked to hear that they think he may have SPD as well. Then our oldest son's new therapist said the same thing. He is not yet officially diagnosed and I'm not sure I agree with that or not as he just seems so different from our first child that it makes me think it may not be true. For now he is still getting therapy anyway as it can't hurt but only help him. I guess time will tell.

2. How has this impacted your child's/family's lives?

With our younger child it's just a matter of a lot of therapy. We have four therapists a week in home and one outside of the house. It's actually nice though because they use play therapy so well they are one on one with him and it allows me to throw on a load of laundry, do dishes and such. With the older one it's harder. As I said before I don't really even believe my younger one has it but with the older one it is easy to see. He gets really frustrated easily and has temper-tantrums multiple times a day. For example if the vacuum is turned on it's too loud for him and he gets really worked up. It's hard to take him to stores because all the lights and sounds really wind him up. Also my children are huge "seekers", they are always looking for proprioceptive input so they can't ever seem to sit still. Because they're so active, it's hard to go places such as out to eat where they are expected to sit still for a time.

3. Do you feel you have a good support system? What could improve a parent's support system?

Actually we just moved for this reason. Our 4 year old was in a bad school district that didn't understand SPD at all. We purposely relocated to get him in a good school district. He has an excellent IEP plan in place with a team that really understands and helps him along the way. We were also lucky to find a great doctor that understands their situation and is great with any referrals we need. And after much searching we were able to find good Occupational Therapists. In our area we even have a library that does SPD book readings once a month where the children have a sensory experience along with the book, and a movie theater that has a sensory friendly movie once a month with the sound turned down, lights left on, and the children are allowed to move around as much as they would like.

4. What has been the best advice and/or treatment you have heard or tried so far?

Finding a good Occupational Therapist in my opinion is the best thing one can do for a sensory child. They can also teach you great ways to keep your child on a "sensory diet" which does wonders to help them throughout the day. Going gluten free and on the Feingold diet (no artificial flavors, colors or preservatives) has really helped also. My best advice is to do what works for your family. In our house, since our children are big seekers we have had a trampoline that took up half our bedroom for them to jump on and an old mattress laid on our couch for them to climb up, roll down, and jump off. Well, most people may think it's a little odd, for us it works to help with their proprioceptive input.

5. What has been the most difficult part of your child's diagnosis and what would make it easier for you?

Other people look at a 4 year old throwing a huge temper-tantrum and assume it is bad parenting. They have no idea that it's their senses being overwhelmed. More public knowledge is crucial for better community support.

6. How has your child's diagnosis affected them/yourself socially and emotionally?

They are such active children I don't have time for myself anymore. I don't even remember who I once was - it really is another life ago. From morning 'til night every day is spent helping my children.

7. Has your child's school been supportive or helpful and how? Do you have 504 plan or IEP?

As mentioned before we have an IEP with an excellent, highly supportive school.

8. Has there been a positive outcome from your child's diagnosis?

I definitely see the world differently. I see other special needs children and people and feel compassion for them more than I ever did before. I also feel so thankful that my children are in fact so high functioning. I'm also extra proud of all their accomplishments as I know how much extra it could be for them to reach them.

9. What would you like the general public to know about this situation?

Not to judge a child's actions by what they see. You may see a child acting wild and throwing a fit in public and the first thing you think of is why can't they control their own kids? But there could be more to the story you don't know.

Of course I could never say for sure what caused the SPD, but one thing I was always suspicious of was when the doctors gave me Pitocin, without my knowledge, when I was in labor. This caused my sons heartbeat to drop dramatically and resulted in an emergency C-section. I just want to say to always make sure you know what your doctors and nurses are giving you and to always question if and why you need it. Also if there is one thing I can't stress enough it's diet. We personally follow the no artificial colors, flavors, or preservatives rule, and any time he has accidently had any of them we have seen a dramatic difference within 24-48 hours that lasts for days. We've made juicing a normal part of our lives as it's a great way to give them extra vitamins and get them used to eating fresh fruits and vegetables.

Also I just wanted to point out it is very common for a child with SPD to have other diagnosis's as well. Our son has also been diagnosed with ADHD, expressive language disorder, and dyspraxia.

Jeanette Baker

Vancouver, British Columbia Canada

1. When did you first notice your child had Sensory Processing Disorder? When and how was he/she officially diagnosed?

I first noticed she had sensory processing disorder when she wouldn't wear any clothes and always wanted to be naked. She would meltdown for hours in the morning because she couldn't get dressed. The tags on her clothes bothered her, she couldn't wear socks or underwear. She didn't like any change in routine and everything always had to be the same. She didn't want to bath/shower, didn't like brushing her teeth/hair, she became agitated easily from too many people speaking at once or too much commotion around her at one time. She also had poor fine motor skills and still does many years later, even writing her name is challenging. She would lose her balance easily and she has always been clumsy. Sleeping has always been difficult for her too.

She is a thrill seeker, always seeking intense quick spinning and moving. She has never been a child to get dizzy and enjoys jumping on the trampoline for hours. She was distracted by sounds and often agitated by several different noises. She loves to chew and lick things from my arm to her fingernails. She reacts negatively to smells and is always blunt with telling others how they smell and that it bothers her. Any environments that are too over stimulating with bright lights or too many colors and sounds cause her to meltdown. We took her to see quite a few different professionals over the years regarding a diagnosis but no one mentioned Sensory Processing Disorder until she was about 8 years old. I took her to see her play therapist and described her daily challenges and she then told me about SPD. (I was so grateful for answers.)

2. How has this impacted your child's/family's lives?

Sensory Processing Disorder has impacted our lives in a huge way. It's been difficult for us to maintain friendships, be more successful in school/career and she has lived in and out of the home on several occasions due to the severity of her meltdowns and behaviors. It has made us see a world that is different. We see everything the way she does now and change things to make it easier for her to cope.

3. Do you feel you have a good support system? What could improve a parent's support system?

I do feel I have a great support system and I have built my life around others who know and understand Sensory Processing Disorder. I am making friends online who have children with similar challenges and seeking others who get it and know what I am going through. I used to be isolated by my child's diagnosis, it is best to find local support groups and friends who will be there for you and not judge your family's situation or how your child is acting.

4. What has been the best advice and/or treatment you have heard or tried so far?

Best advice – "You have not failed! You have just tried 10,000 things that haven't worked". We have learned to celebrate the small things as they truly are the big things. One day at a time. We do everything at her pace now. I have learned acceptance. I have learned patience. Educate and advocate. Read as much as I could so I could be the voice my child needed me to be for her. Best treatment - a lot of love and understanding. Brushing and joint compressions have been a life saver for us. Pressure vests and weighted therapy.

5. What has been the most difficult part of your child's diagnosis and what would make it easier for you?

The most difficult part of her diagnosis has been lack of sleep, constant meltdowns, lack of services, unsupportive schooling, medication pressure and watching her suffer with the daily issues she struggles with the most. I think the way to improve it would be for teachers/schools and the general public to be more educated about SPD, more services for her to learn different ways to cope with SPD, easier access to Occupational Therapy and therapy items, ways for me to learn how to help her more and have others around me know and understand SPD. Parenting courses that aren't for regular children without a diagnosis and meant for parents who have children with a different diagnosis.

6. How has your child's diagnosis affected them/yourself socially and emotionally?

For her socially, it has been difficult to maintain healthy friendships. She plays a lot on her own or with children younger than herself. Emotionally for her she is often impulsive, easily frustrated and her moods can change quickly, causing huge outbursts. She is more successful in a small group setting or one on one. Her diagnosis has affected me socially as I do not have time to be as social as I once was. I don't have much time for friends and it is difficult finding friends who are accepting of her diagnosis, people who aren't judging and making hurtful comments about her behavior. Emotionally for me, it has been very tough. I get sad a lot. I have cried so much as it has been tougher than I could ever have imagined possible. I have felt hopeless for many years, nothing worked and it kept getting worse and worse and totally out of my control. I didn't know what else to try or do, I also felt I was a failing mom and she'd be better off without me. My heart has broken a million times, I've shed millions of tears and I've broken down.

I am finally feeling some success. We have bad days but they are getting better.

7. Has your child's school been supportive or helpful and how? Do you have 504 plan or IEP?

We have had a couple of supportive schools but we have had really unsupportive schools too. We do have IEP in place but her schools always give her work she was capable of doing many years before. It is too easy and not challenging enough to teach her anything new. She goes just for a couple of hours a day. She has always had teachers' aides to assist her in daily school work and activities. I don't feel they try hard enough to give her the proper education she deserves. Every year I feel she is passed from one grade to the next when she has not been given the time or work to properly be ready for the next school year. After several years she has now fallen behind the other children in her grade level.

8. Has there been a positive outcome from your child's diagnosis?

Things are improving for her as she gets older. She is becoming more social, recognizing feelings and emotions better. She has learned better self-regulation skills and to appreciate her successes. It has made our relationship stronger. We work on everything together. We are a team. I have learned how to be a better parent and I am grateful that she is my daughter and I am her mom. I wouldn't have it any other way. Special children are given to special parents. I have become her advocate and her voice at times when I didn't think I ever could. It has made us both stronger.

9. What would you like the general public to know about this situation?

Being a child with Sensory Processing Disorder is very challenging. They need to work so much harder than others do to get through each day and nothing comes easy for them. Each day brings new struggles and most events in their lives can be difficult. Each child has their own differences, all children with Sensory Processing Disorder are different. They all see and feel everything differently to others. Being a parent of a child with Sensory Processing Disorder is really tough. You learn everything as you go, everything is trial and error. Trying to find the things that work for your child, what doesn't work, and keeping on the same schedule all the time can be extremely hard on a parent.

10. If there is anything else you would like to share with our readers on the subject, not included above, please add it here.

Juggling careers, school, relationships, therapy appointments, school meetings, medical bills, paying for therapy items, doing research and coping with your child's behaviors every day is stressful. Sensory parents have several extra worries, chores and errands to do every day. When you see a sensory parent who is having a tough time, or a sensory child, reach out, give a hug or a hand to help. They don't need judgments, they need help sometimes too. Be a support for them.

Erica Cornell

Oil City,Pa

1. When did you first notice your child had Sensory Processing Disorder? When and how was he/she officially diagnosed?

I noticed when he was about 3 years old that something wasn't right and I was tired of hearing he was a typical boy. He wasn't diagnosed until he was 7.

2. How has this impacted your child's/family's lives?

It's hard for him to deal with all the sensations he doesn't understand. He has a lot of tantrums still.

3. Do you feel you have a good support system? What could improve a parent's support system?

My family is the only support we have in our area. There really aren't any groups in the area.

4. What has been the best advice and/or treatment you have heard or tried so far?

We do OT and that seems to help some. We have incorporated certain therapy methods at home as well.

5. What has been the most difficult part of your child's diagnosis and what would make it easier for you?

The fact that a lot of people still don't know what SPD is. More education would be so much more helpful.

6. How has your child's diagnosis affected them/yourself socially and emotionally?

He has very poor social skills and it has hurt him since the other kids don't understand, they pick on him.

7. Has your child's school been supportive or helpful and how? Do you have 504 plan or IEP?

The school really hasn't been that supportive. I tried for an IEP and was denied because he is "too smart".

8. Has there been a positive outcome from your child's diagnosis?

Yes, we finally know what we are dealing with and how we can help him.

9. What would you like the general public to know about this situation?

These aren't bad kids or bad parenting. They are children who interpret everything differently and don't understand why.

10. If there is anything else you would like to share with our readers on the subject, not included above, please add it here.

Morgan L Masterson

Colorado Springs, USA

1. When did you first notice your child had Sensory Processing Disorder? When and how was he/she officially diagnosed?

When she was about 2 years old, maybe 2½. She showed a lot of obsessive behaviors and anxieties, and was very active and clumsy. She was diagnosed when she was about 3½ after seeing a child psychologist, an OT and PT. Psychologist suspected it, OT confirmed it.

2. How has this impacted your child's/family's lives?

We have a lot of appointments now. But we are learning ways to calm her anxieties and help her satisfy her seeking behavior.

3. Do you feel you have a good support system? What could improve a parent's support system?

I do feel like I have a good support system. Improvements could be made in awareness, so people don't' just think we can't control our kid.

4. What has been the best advice and/or treatment you have heard or tried so far?

Brushing! And be patient, she can't help herself.

5. What has been the most difficult part of your child's diagnosis and what would make it easier for you?

6. How has your child's diagnosis affected them/yourself socially and emotionally?

Not at all. Our lives are a little more busy with doctors' appointments, but we meet new people.

7. Has your child's school been supportive or helpful and how? Do you have

504 plan or IEP?

She's not in school yet.

8. Has there been a positive outcome from your child's diagnosis?

Lots of new things learned every week. And tips to use on my younger child as well.

9. What would you like the general public to know about this situation?

Kids can't help it! They aren't out of control or bad kids, they just have different thoughts and actions than others.   My daughter is very impulsive. She doesn't do things to be "bad" she just needs sensory input constantly.

10. If there is anything else you would like to share with our readers on the

subject, not included above, please add it here.

Be patient! If you see a kid out in public throwing a fit or having a meltdown, don't just assume the child is a brat. Every kid is different, and sometimes the smallest thing can cause a meltdown for an SPD kiddo. It's not the kid's fault. Don't judge the child or the parents!

Shannon Bussells

Lexington USA

1. *When did you first notice your child had Sensory Processing Disorder? When and how was he/she officially diagnosed?*

My son Chase has had sensory problems since birth. But I was completely unaware of this disorder and knew nothing about it until I took him to his first speech evaluation through a speech therapist at my local hospital. She is the one who told me he had it. He was not officially diagnosed with it until this year (2013) at the age of 4 by an Occupational Therapist.

2. *How has this impacted your child's/family's lives?*

It has affected our whole family tremendously as we thought he had Autism or ASD. I have spent two years of my life dedicated to getting him tested by everybody possible. He's been tested by the schools all the way to a developmental pediatrician. I have spent the past two years dedicated to his needs and having to re-teach him basic life skills such as getting dressed on his own every day. His memory for these types of skills is very short term. It takes months to teach him one skill at a time.

3. *Do you feel you have a good support system? What could improve a parent's support system?*

I personally do not have a good support system at all. I have had to fight with my own family all these years that he has a problem and is not just a spoiled brat suffering from middle child syndrome. I suggest that other parents: 1) find all the support they can online or otherwise because it is very draining emotionally and physically; and 2) if you are a mother like me, being told it's just me or my fault, follow your gut feeling. Mothers' intuition won't ever let you down!

4. What has been the best advice and/or treatment you have heard or tried

so far?

The only thing I have been told is to keep taking him to speech and occupational therapy. And I have finally found an organization that is working wonders for him. Best advice is - be persistent.

5. What has been the most difficult part of your child's diagnosis and what

would make it easier for you?

I am still uneducated about his disorder and trying to learn all that I can. It's been hard trying to understand everything. I have been given a list of suggested books to read, but I am unable to do so. I cannot focus enough to read books.

6. How has your child's diagnosis affected them/yourself socially

and emotionally?

Socially; he has no friends because of this. Other kids cannot understand him verbally and he would rather play alone. His SPD stops him from being able to cope well in crowds.

Emotionally; it's a very hard thing to cope with. His meltdowns and inability to problem-solve keeps me stressed out. He cries and gets angry instead of trying to figure things out on his own. He used to use anger and violence when he got frustrated. But now he just cries and throws fits.

7. Has your child's school been supportive or helpful and how? Do you have

504 plan or IEP?

I do have an IEP plan but it's only for speech delay. He is not in school yet, but we are hoping for him to be accepted into PreK this year.

8. Has there been a positive outcome from your child's diagnosis?

Yes. Being diagnosed is what got him his acceptance into Occupational Therapy. He has taken huge strides in the past 2 months or so that he has been going. I have found out that one of his biggest problems is his reaction to noises. I knew he didn't like loud noises, but I never knew it affected him in little things like play as well.

9. What would you like the general public to know about this situation?

When you see a child having a meltdown or what looks like a "temper tantrum", ask the parents about that child before assuming they are just a spoiled brat not getting their way.

10. If there is anything else you would like to share with our readers on the subject, not included above, please add it here.

I don't have anything else as of right now because I am still learning myself.

Kristen S.

Rexburg, Madison

1. *When did you first notice your child had Sensory Processing Disorder? When and how was he/she officially diagnosed?*

As a young infant he would sit for hours just watching the ceiling fan go round-and-round. His favorite toy was the top of another toy. A palm tree with leaves that spun. He doesn't roll cars on the floor, he turns them on their roof and spins them. If it spins, he'll find a way to make it happen.

I first took him for evaluation shortly after he was 2 years old. We were at a grandparent's home with a rock gravel driveway. He sat for nearly 4 hours throwing those rocks. Didn't move or say anything. This seemed unusual to me - that a 2 year old would do this!

My son is 5 and still hasn't been officially diagnosed. The doctors and therapists say he doesn't have enough of one thing to make a concrete diagnosis. And he's so young it will change anyway.

2. *How has this impacted your child's/family's lives?*

My son Kaleb is the oldest. His brother is only 14 months younger. Kaleb has Speech, Occupational, and Physical therapy every week, one hour sessions each. It has been hard on his younger brother. All little brother sees is that big brother gets to go play and he wants to go too! It has taken an emotional and physical toll as we've struggled to balance therapy appointments and two younger kids. We can't be spontaneous. Everything has to be planned out and pre-discussed days in advance. Several times we've had to quickly leave a park, party, restaurant or store when things were too much to handle and a severe meltdown was imminent. Even if the other kids or mom and dad are still having fun we have to focus on Kaleb and what he needs.

3. Do you feel you have a good support system? What could improve a parent's support system?

I am still learning what support there is all around me. I have found valuable help in online communities. The therapists have been helpful in teaching me how I can best help Kaleb not only learn and grow, but thrive.

I wish I could find a physical parent support group where our kids could get together for playdates and we could lean on each other for support and help.

4. What has been the best advice and/or treatment you have heard or tried so far?

With my son it has been to not yell. Yelling makes things worse. I have to get down on his level and quietly ask him why he is acting this way and what he is feeling.

5. What has been the most difficult part of your child's diagnosis and what would make it easier for you?

The hardest part has been learning what I need to do to help my son thrive and not get left behind.

Of course it would be easier if my son acted like his two other cousins that were all born within a few weeks of each other. But we are here so it would be nice if the schools and doctors knew more and were able to help guide me through this scary maze of upcoming school.

6. How has your child's diagnosis affected them/yourself socially and emotionally?

My son is a watcher. He watches and laughs as kids slide down slides or have fun. It makes me feel sad that he doesn't have friends, that he doesn't want to run and play and laugh with peers. It affects him emotionally because he doesn't voice out loud that he wants or needs attention. Sometimes I get focused on other kids or tasks and forget to sit down and play quietly with my son, who is also craving attention but isn't vocal about it.

7. Has your child's school been supportive or helpful and how? Do you have 504 plan or IEP?

School has been so-so. We had a wonderful IEP when he started preschool. The teachers kept me informed what each day was like and how his progress was. Kaleb will be starting Kindergarten soon and so far it hasn't been too positive. We had the IEP 3 months ago and I never received a copy of it. I tried to call and get hold of the teacher to get help with some suggestions from the OT. I finally got through to the district only to be told the school is shut down until back-to-school night and there's nothing they can do.

8. Has there been a positive outcome from your child's diagnosis?

That we are aware of it and we have been able to get him so much help. I have also learned to be a calmer and more understanding parent.

9. What would you like the general public to know about this situation?

10. If there is anything else you would like to share with our readers on the subject, not included above, please add it here.

Christie Spence
Canadian Texas, USA

1. When did you first notice your child had Sensory Processing Disorder? When and how was he/she officially diagnosed?

At age 18 months, he had delays and a food aversion. We saw ECI for the delays but at age 2½ he began having some "what looked like behavioral problems". We had him evaluated at 3 years old. Sure enough - SPD.

2. How has this impacted your child's/family's lives?

It has impacted us dramatically. All of our energy and focus is to "help" him cope and teach him to communicate and avoid meltdowns.

3. Do you feel you have a good support system? What could improve a parent's support system?

Yes, I have a great support system. The only thing I would hope to improve is the world's understanding and involvement in the treatment plans for these kids.

4. What has been the best advice and/or treatment you have heard or tried so far?

Be consistent. Be understanding. He is not "giving" you a hard time…. he is "having" a hard time.

5. What has been the most difficult part of your child's diagnosis and what would make it easier for you?

The most difficult part is the anxiety he has with change. And the fact that we can't have a spur of the moment change in plans. Everything has to be planned and prepared for, along with a packed bag with "things" he may need while we are out (Neoprene vest, fidgets, train toys, ear protectors, iPad).

6. How has your child's diagnosis affected them/yourself socially and emotionally?

My child's diagnosis has turned me into a walking/talking therapist. I can no longer have a normal mommy conversation with another parent at the park bench. I feel like I have to make every moment count. Every chance I get, I have to be "interacting with" or helping him communicate better. Early intervention is so important they say. So, I feel that, at 3 years old, this is the time he needs the most from me. I am saving his life right now. No time for petty talk. I have to help my son.

7. Has your child's school been supportive or helpful and how? Do you have 504 plan or IEP?

We are not in the school system yet. He goes for evaluation on September 25th. He is 3 years old. Currently SPD is not in the DSM-5 as a "stand alone" diagnosis. So, I pray that the therapist will have a "good day" and say that we qualify for services just based on his delays. I'm nervous about the school system's knowledge of SPD in the first place. Do they know what it is? Do they treat any other children with it? How do they handle them? What amount of therapy will they get? Speech? Occupational? I just worry, worry, worry.

8. Has there been a positive outcome from your child's diagnosis?

The diagnosis itself has been a positive for us, simply because we know how to treat it! We know what it is! Before, we knew something was going on…. we just didn't know what, or how to fix it. A diagnosis gave us a plan and some hope.

9. What would you like the general public to know about this situation?

These babies have to deal with so much! Their little neurological systems are all mixed up. That's hard to deal with in itself. Next, you don't know how to cope, so you act out. When you act out, your parents are angry. Now they feel sad because their parents are angry and upset with them. They don't know how to cope with that pain either, so they melt. These kids need understanding and help learning how to cope with their anxieties and feelings. As a parent or teacher or therapist, it is tiring. It is hard. It is emotionally draining. But don't give up! The things you say and do, will either help him or hurt him. You hold the key.

10. *If there is anything else you would like to share with our readers on the subject, not included above, please add it here.*

Angela Slate

Duncan, OK, USA

1. When did you first notice your child had Sensory Processing Disorder? When and how was he/she officially diagnosed?

Cooper started screaming when he was 2 years old and has never stopped being loud. Cooper was diagnosed at age 22 months, firstly by the SSI's physiologist then by Sooner Start, our Oklahoma program for kids with autism and other developmental disorders.

2. How has this impacted your child's/family's lives?

It's been rough, Cooper is self-abusive, and to others also. Meltdowns are so tough he has no knowledge of when he hurts himself in one. My 6 year old will tell you, "My brother screams all the time, and sometimes I need a break because he can be mean to me". It's not all bad though, Cooper at times can be perfect.

3. Do you feel you have a good support system? What could improve a parent's support system?

Yes, I'm very happy with my Facebook support groups, his OT and our family.

4. What has been the best advice and/or treatment you have heard or tried so far?

Just to be consistent in what you do.

5. What has been the most difficult part of your child's diagnosis and what would make it easier for you?

That they can't do anything to really help him, he can't sleep, and sometimes it just seems like he's in pain.

6. How has your child's diagnosis affected them/yourself socially

and emotionally?

We can't go out in public, he can't handle going out to eat or even going to his brother's soccer games.

7. Has your child's school been supportive or helpful and how? Do you have

504 plan or IEP?

Since Cooper is so young he has an IFSP. We've got him in to special program for young disabled children.

8. Has there been a positive outcome from your child's diagnosis?

Yes, I am able to get him what help I can, and we are trying visual schedules. We've accomplished some small tasks.

9. What would you like the general public to know about this situation?

That it is hard to have a special needs child, but that you can do it. There are wonderful moments, and there are times when you want to pull your hair out. They are still little people who need lots of love, and lots of direction. Keep the faith, study as much as you can. Talk to friends and family about your child's condition, find a great doctor and support team.

10. If there is anything else you would like to share with our readers on the

subject, not included above, please add it here.

Marzena Walker

Plainfield, IL, USA

1. When did you first notice your child had Sensory Processing Disorder? When and how was he/she officially diagnosed?

My son has Dyspraxia and three different vision processing disorders. I've always known that my son was different. He had so many great qualities and so many strange things that he did or struggled with. He was diagnosed at 7 years old and has just turned 8. My son had completed first grade. He struggled in pre-school, kindergarten and first grade. The teachers kept telling me that he was a little behind but that he would catch up. The second half of first grade was so tough for him. He was very aware of the fact that other kids were ahead of where he was. We practiced and practiced at home and made small gains, but his friends were making leaps ahead. I talked to several people at the school (also a pediatrician) struggling to find out if there was someone that could help us, or if should have him assessed by some type of specialist. Everyone kept saying he would grow out of it and I had to keep working with him. The school recommended that he go on to second grade.

Over the summer, we wanted to get him more help so we took him to three different learning centers to help with his writing and reading. Each one without knowing what the other said told us that he was at a pre-school reading level (even though he was about to go into second grade). Coincidentally, my younger son broke his arm and I asked his pediatric orthopedic for help since I knew my older guy struggled with fine motor skills and thought that maybe this doctor could help. He told me about a pediatric therapy place. The therapist was great. The day that she assessed him she told us about Sensory Processing Disorder and dyspraxia and laid out a therapy plan. She also was concerned about his vision processing. A developmental optometrist later diagnosed him with three different vision processing disorders even though he has 20/20 vision medically. He has completed first grade again and seems to be retaining most of what he learned. He is reading better and faster than he did a couple of months ago.

I went back to the school armed with the information from the learning center assessments and report from the therapist. After talking, screaming and crying in the principal's office, he finally agreed to hold my son back and have him repeat first grade. He really needed the extra year to address the fine motor skills, core trunk muscles, motor planning and vision processing.

For our family, I describe it as organized chaos. Both my husband and I work and we have three boys (8, 4 and 2 years old). My oldest goes to vision therapy one day a week, we do half an hour of home based vision therapy every day, he goes for occupational therapy one day a week and we do daily activities to help him build his muscles and stay regulated. He has started doing horseback riding once a week to help with his anxiety and build core muscles, he has piano lessons, does a social skills class weekly and sees a psychologist weekly. My younger two also are doing weekly occupational therapy as I highly suspect that they have some sensory processing issues. With all this, I feel like this is helping and while it is chaotic, I can see the way that these things help them.

3. Do you feel you have a good support system? What could improve a

parent's support system?

Not really. I feel like we keep stumbling onto what could help our boys. I'm learning that there is some information out there but I still get very overwhelmed with not knowing if we are doing the right things at the right time. I wish that there was a person or doctor that I could find that had a lot of knowledge and experience with this. I feel like I'm doing more educating now than them. I need someone to help me sort through potential solutions and develop actions plans that I can implement for my sons (all three) on a daily basis. I've learned a lot from the couple of parent support groups on Facebook but it would be nice to talk to knowledgeable people face to face about this.

Our OT is great but I want more linkage between medical, vision, occupational therapy and psychology. Also, a professional that can better help with making sure we eliminate the bad foods from my boys' diet and take the right supplements/vitamins, etc. But most of all, I need help making the school system understand his needs and how best to help him. I don't want to be told that he is not holding himself accountable for things that he struggles with. I don't want to be arguing about why my son needs to sit facing the front of the classroom and why he needs frequent movement breaks. I want the teachers to understand this enough so that when they come to me with a problem they can offer things that we can try to help with the problem - not just tell me to talk to the other professionals that my son deals with. The worst was when the teacher tried to suggest that maybe medication would help my son.

He works harder than any of his peers and while his successes are not as big as theirs, he gives 150% every day. He wants to please everyone and it breaks my heart to see him feel and think that he is constantly letting them down by not catching on as fast. Why shouldn't the schools and teachers work just as hard for him as he does for them? Don't get me wrong, they try but are not trying as hard as he is.

4. *What has been the best advice and/or treatment you have heard or tried so far?*

Occupational therapy has helped tremendously with fine motor skills, core trunk muscles and motor planning. Vision therapy is unbelievable. His reading and writing are improving weekly as a result of all the hard work on the daily vision therapy. Therapeutic listening therapy really seems to help him feel calm and regulated. Horseback riding is great for muscles and motor planning and helping with anxiety as he learns to control such a large animal (best part - he thinks he is doing this just for fun). Social skills class to help him better understand the reactions of others and not take so personally everything that everyone else says and does (he too desperately wants to be everyone's friend). He just started a probiotic and fish oil supplement and we hope these work wonders. Also, we have eliminated most food dyes (especially red 40).

5. What has been the most difficult part of your child's diagnosis and what would make it easier for you?

Most difficult part is understanding the best way to help him and helping school and family also understand. More awareness would make it easier. When I say SPD and dyspraxia, most people look at me like I'm making it up.

6. How has your child's diagnosis affected them/yourself socially and emotionally?

I feel emotionally drained. I hope that we are doing the right things for him but know that as he gets older, we will have different challenges to deal with. This scares me as I'm a planner. I can't plan what I don't know yet. I feel like there is still so much that I should but don't know yet. Only my parents can watch my kids. We have tried but had no luck yet to find a sitter who can handle the boys and who they would be comfortable with. We both work and unless the boys come with us, we go nowhere else. Unfortunately, I have not yet found a way to not work as I'm the primary financial contributor to our family. I get so overwhelmed with the need to work and the desire to try to spend as much time with the boys as I can to help them.

7. Has your child's school been supportive or helpful and how? Do you have 504 plan or IEP?

My son's school tried to convince me that a 504 plan would be sufficient, even though we decided to have him repeat first grade. I refused and eventually got them to accept doing an IEP. This was great. This also was when I was just starting to learn about SPD and dyspraxia and know that the IEP could have been better. I'll work on making sure that it is for this upcoming school year. My son goes for special education for reading and his regular class for all other activities. He also sees an OT at school for half an hour a week. Both of these have helped tremendously. Otherwise, it seems like whenever I bring a new idea to them, it takes a lot of convincing to get them to try it. My biggest concern is that no one at that school, with maybe the exception of the OT, knows anything about his disorders.

8. *Has there been a positive outcome from your child's diagnosis?*

Yes. I feel like we are finally understanding him and are able to find things that can help him be successful and feel good about himself. I cried when I read the first few chapters of *Out of Sync Child* after my son was diagnosed. It explained so much about the things that he can and cannot do or why he does them. I felt like, for the first time, I was not just imagining things. There were other kids and families dealing with the same situations as we were. I've always felt that information was power. My son is too young to obtain and use that information but I can help him be a happy and successful person.

9. *What would you like the general public to know about this situation?*

There are so many with this disorder and while there are similarities between people with the disorder, each person is different. This "blind" disorder is a real disorder. Real things can be done and should be done to help people with this disorder so that they can become highly functioning adults and contribute to society. Kids can't always tell you that there is something wrong, especially when they were born with these disorders. People need to know. Educators need to know and speak up. Pediatricians need to know. I look at my extended family and know that many of them have struggled in life because no one knew why they were the way they were, and why they did things differently to everyone else.   So much could have been done for them. Real understanding is the solution.

10. *If there is anything else you would like to share with our readers on the subject, not included above, please add it here.*

No.

Sharon Walsh

Dublin, Ireland

1. When did you first notice your child had Sensory Processing Disorder? When and how was he/she officially diagnosed?

Our lady was always quirky, but whenever we mentioned it to a GP or nurse we were told no two kids are the same. But when her school report came back to us in 2012 we investigated ourselves. She was officially diagnosed in December 2012 by an OT. We also found she has a specific language delay.

2. How has this impacted your child's/family's lives?

It's a huge impact as our eldest doesn't understand how little things like having a shower can set off an hour long meltdown. She also gets less time and attention because of appointments. When we are going to a party both my husband and I need to go so if she kicks off one can leave. Our youngest, who's two, now copies the behavior and we find ourselves watching to see if it's terrible twos or SPD.

3. Do you feel you have a good support system? What could improve a parent's support system?

We have NO support from our government. She is not bad enough to receive help because she can tie a lace, even though it comes undone after a couple of minutes. We have to pay privately for an OT and an osteopath weekly. I think all children with a diagnosed hardship should receive treatment even at a reduced cost in the public system.

4. What has been the best advice and/or treatment you have heard or tried so far?

To speak calmly to her. If I shout she panics and has a major meltdown. Warn her in advance of any change to routine or event coming up. It gives her time to process. We also tell her to just squeeze our hands if she's feeling overwhelmed.

5. What has been the most difficult part of your child's diagnosis and what would make it easier for you?

The difficulty we have is getting support from our government body. It seems like we work to pay her OT costs.

6. How has your child's diagnosis affected them/yourself socially and emotionally?

It makes us weary when there's an event/party coming up - we get anxious as to how she will handle the situation. She gets anxious too, picks her nails, and sweats profusely. Sometimes she just cries.

7. Has your child's school been supportive or helpful and how? Do you have 504 plan or IEP?

School is very helpful but can't offer any support service.

8. Has there been a positive outcome from your child's diagnosis?

Yes. We now understand her quirks are a nervous reaction to a situation or nerves. We can now try prevent a meltdown by giving notice in preparation for something coming up. When she kicks off because she doesn't want a shower we tell her we know she doesn't like it, we know it hurts her and takes too long. Before we knew how hard it was for her, we would just get her out of the shower and punish her by taking something away.

9. What would you like the general public to know about this situation?

I'm not a bad parent! She's not a bad child!

She finds life hard, even the general things we take for granted.

She gets hurt easier when playing, she's not a cry baby!

*10. **If there is anything else you would like to share with our readers on the subject, not included above, please add it here.**

It's extremely hard, time consuming and fearful having a child with anything wrong. But it's most rewarding when my girl has a shower without tears, or when she comes home with a new reading book from school.

There will always be people who judge..... let them! You know how awesome your kiddos are because of everything they do...

Karly Montsion

Cary, IL

1. When did you first notice your child had Sensory Processing Disorder? When and how was he/she officially diagnosed?

I had been in and out of the pediatrician's office for over two years. It started with sleep issues. My daughter would not sleep through the night for anything. I would rock her and she would be fine, but the minute I put her back in her bed she would scream like someone was pulling her toenails out. It was hard and we were so sleep-deprived. Eventually my husband blew up an air mattress and slept on the floor in her room with her and that helped. We also had several behavioral issues. My daughter would pull her own hair out, bite herself and smack herself on the head when she was frustrated or angry. She would bang her head against the wall and throw massive screaming tantrums. She would not sit still and would repeat herself over and over. Her emotions were always over exaggerated.

We've seen our regular doctor, a behavioral specialist and allergists. I finally realized my regular pediatrician wasn't helping us work toward a diagnosis and was only running tests and looking into things that I pushed her to look into. I switched pediatricians in June and immediately received a diagnosis and an evaluation request for OT. We have seen SIGNIFICANT improvements since we've started OT. I sometimes kick myself for not switching doctors sooner!

2. How has this impacted your child's/family's lives?

Pre diagnosis, it was terribly hard. Our patience was running so thin, having two other children. We would yell a lot and get to the point where we were short with all the children. We were run ragged and we were all suffering. Post diagnosis things are improving. We still have our challenges and are learning every day but now that we know HOW to go about things, there seems to be more of a flow in family time. Everyone is more comfortable hanging around each other and things seem a bit calmer.

3. Do you feel you have a good support system? What could improve a parent's support system?

I have a good support system – just not all of our family. Some don't "see" what we see and don't believe there is anything going on. Most of our family supports us and helps out where they can. I have an amazing support system with our friends and social media and that certainly helps. I think support would be easier to come by if SPD was more widely known. I hadn't even heard about it until we received our diagnosis. I'm doing my best to spread the word and talk to anyone who will listen!

4. What has been the best advice and/or treatment you have heard or tried so far?

OT has definitely been wonderful. I have seen progress with our daughter and her therapist put her hand on my shoulder one day and looked me square in the eyes. She said to me, "If you're already seeing results this early it means that you're doing something right. You're taking what I'm teaching you and applying it at home. These changes are because of you." I almost cried right there. It was the encouragement I needed to keep working on it because some days it really is just hard…

5. What has been the most difficult part of your child's diagnosis and what would make it easier for you?

The most difficult is that it's something that not everyone sees. It's hard to get some parents to understand that my daughter isn't pushing and hitting your child because she's intentionally trying to be mean (though at 3 years old, sometimes it is). It's hard for them to understand that I can't always just "get her under control" or "take care of it".

6. How has your child's diagnosis affected them/yourself socially

and emotionally?

I think it has affected her in a great way! Now that we have a diagnosis and know what we're working with, it's easier for her to be friendly to other people because we work so hard on keeping her body regulated. For me, I'd say it's mostly emotionally. I feel relief knowing there is an answer and knowing that we can work toward keeping her SPD under control. I know how to talk to her teachers in the future and let them know what's going on.

7. Has your child's school been supportive or helpful and how? Do you have

504 plan or IEP?

My daughter will start preschool in a few weeks and I am waiting on her class information so that I can talk to her teachers. This answer has to be N/A for now.

8. Has there been a positive outcome from your child's diagnosis?

Yes! Lots of improvement with OT! Sleep issues had been mostly resolved pre diagnosis but since diagnosis and therapy, she will sleep longer and get better sleep cycles.

9. What would you like the general public to know about this situation?

That it is REAL and parents like me need your support. We need your patience and your understanding. Until you've walked a mile in our shoes, please don't assume we don't know how to handle our children and please don't jump to the conclusion that our children are "bad" because they're not. They're loving and affectionate and wanted to be treated like every other child on the face of the planet.

One resolution that did help with us was cutting dairy out of my daughter's diet. She was allergy tested by three different allergists but her scratch tests always came back negative. Since most allergists only test blood by IgG tests, those were negative too. We found a doctor that would run an IgE test (which isn't trusted by the allergy association) and her responsive levels were ridiculously high. Since cutting dairy out of her diet, her tantrums have been more manageable, her sleep has been better (her sleep started improving once we figured this out) and she has been better able to focus on things. If you'd like more information (I feel like I can talk about this for hours) please let me know and I am happy to dive deeper with you.

Sherry Johnstone

Burlington U.S.A.

1. When did you first notice your child had Sensory Processing Disorder? When and how was he/she officially diagnosed?

I noticed that my child had sensory issues at 18 months. He was diagnosed at age 2 by Early Intervention specialists.

2. How has this impacted your child's/family's lives?

There is no set daily routine in our household. Things change "on the fly", depending on my child's needs on any given day (and some days they change hour to hour).

3. Do you feel you have a good support system? What could improve a parent's support system?

We are fortunate to have the support of his school and his developmental pediatrician. There is no family support.

4. What has been the best advice and/or treatment you have heard or tried so far?

The therapies that helped my child the most were OT, speech therapy and behavioral therapy.

5. What has been the most difficult part of your child's diagnosis and what would make it easier for you?

The difficult part for me is seeing him struggle with social situations and making friends. We have done everything we can to help him be successful in his interactions with other children, but it is ultimately up to him to keep the friendships going.

6. How has your child's diagnosis affected them/yourself socially

and emotionally?

My husband and I have no social life. There are no sitters available that can handle my child's needs. We have no family members that will help.

7. Has your child's school been supportive or helpful and how? Do you have

504 plan or IEP?

My child's school has been very accommodating. He has had an IEP since preschool (he will be entering Grade 2 in the fall).

8. Has there been a positive outcome from your child's diagnosis?

Because of all the therapies he received at such a young age, many of his issues are much improved. Some he has outgrown or learned to handle better.

9. What would you like the general public to know about this situation?

That Sensory Processing Disorder can be managed with interventions and therapies tailored to your child's needs.

10. If there is anything else you would like to share with our readers on the

subject, not included above, please add it here.

Ronetta Fosnaugh

Cedarville, Ohio USA

1. When did you first notice your child had Sensory Processing Disorder? When and how was he/she officially diagnosed?

Patience was 5 months old when we knew something was wrong. She was actually 14 months old when she was diagnosed through developmental pediatrics at the Children's Hospital.

2. How has this impacted your child's/family's lives?

Lots of therapy, lots of living adjustments, temperature adjustments, meal time adjustments, sensory equipment and how aids for daily living are done.

3. Do you feel you have a good support system? What could improve a parent's support system?

My family is great support, *Help Me Grow* is a great resource for under 3 year olds, I have a couple of friends that I work with who also have sensory/autistic children, but I have really enjoyed the support group online.

4. What has been the best advice and/or treatment you have heard or tried so far?

I would have to say the weighted vests/blankets have helped the most, of course all of the therapies help also.

5. What has been the most difficult part of your child's diagnosis and what would make it easier for you?

Knowing that her life is always going to be difficult and I can't change that, but finding out there is a lot of help out there if you seek it out. It would have been great if when she was diagnosed the doctor's office had offered information about the disease and where to get help.

6. How has your child's diagnosis affected them/yourself socially and emotionally?

Fortunately I am not concerned about what people think, but words are really harsh. I just wish people would ask, rather than assume, what is wrong - instead of telling me to get a handle on my kid.

7. Has your child's school been supportive or helpful and how? Do you have 504 plan or IEP?

The school didn't take us seriously at first. We had to get loud that we were not going to stand for anything less that the care she gets with us and her therapy. They have got her on an IEP, but we're still fighting for a 504 plan.

8. Has there been a positive outcome from your child's diagnosis?

I have been able to make people in the public more aware of sensory processing disorders/autism spectrum disorders, and knowledge is power.

9. What would you like the general public to know about this situation?

That these kids are not brats, spoiled, or out of control. This is a serious illness with life-altering consequences.

10. If there is anything else you would like to share with our readers on the subject, not included above, please add it here.

We love our children without reservation, good day or bad, hitting, biting, spitting, cursing, and anything else their little minds can imagine. It is not always easy, but worth it all the same. Please don't judge us for what you think you know, ask me.

Lila Lins

Moose Jaw, Canada

1. *When did you first notice your child had Sensory Processing Disorder?*
When and how was he/she officially diagnosed?

It took us a little longer to realize it because she was diagnosed with only 60% hearing at 2½ years old. Within 8 months after that we realized that lack of hearing wasn't all that made her different from other kids the same age. She was just diagnosed at 3½ years of age, July 22, 2013.

2. *How has this impacted your child's/family's lives?*

Before the diagnosis we were short with her, frustrated, constantly questioned ourselves as parents and wondered why she was so different from other children her own age. Not to mention I was tired of other parents judging us negatively. Now that we have an answer we feel relief, we want to learn all we can about her disorder, how we can help her so school and socializing won't be so hard for her.

3. *Do you feel you have a good support system? What could improve a*
parent's support system?

My husband's parents and mine are a tremendous help financially, emotionally and physically (when we need a break from the constant energy). Also she is in a daycare and the daycare owner is amazing with our daughter and constantly offers to help in any way she can. I do feel like my daughter's doctor reacted negatively when I told him that she was seeing therapists and specialists to rule out or diagnose any mental disorders. His response was simply "she's a little girl, if she's not energetic I'd be concerned". I wish the doctor would realize that we are concerned for her health and safety, she takes dangerous risks daily with no fear at all.

4. What has been the best advice and/or treatment you have heard or tried so far?

Sitting calmly on the couch with her wrapped tightly in a blanket in my arms, the compression seems to calm her down

5. What has been the most difficult part of your child's diagnosis and what would make it easier for you?

The lack of support from her doctor, we are considering taking her to my family doctor and hoping for a more open mind.

6. How has your child's diagnosis affected them/yourself socially and emotionally?

We feel relief, we have an answer, close family and friends are all so supportive. We are way more patient with her because we know she's just a little different than other children her age. Already we see a change in her, we offer more praise and less negative reaction.

7. Has your child's school been supportive or helpful and how? Do you have 504 plan or IEP?

She's not in school yet, however the daycare is incredible. We were told by the therapist that we have a year to help her and figure out what works for our daughter because when she goes to school they can't see her anymore unless I make it very clear that she absolutely needs their help.

8. Has there been a positive outcome from your child's diagnosis?

We're more patient with her and understanding.

9. What would you like the general public to know about this situation?

That kids like her are not just "wild and out of control" that they are just a little different to their peers.

I wish people knew more about this disorder. When you mention mental
disabilities or disorders people automatically jump to ADD or ADHD, and
I wish people knew that there are other disorders and they aren't any less
important.

Jax

Swift Current, SK Canada

1. When did you first notice your child had Sensory Processing Disorder? When and how was he/she officially diagnosed?

Around the age of 2½ years, we noticed that our daughter had some differences but she was our oldest and honestly, we didn't know. Friends would say she was fine. We found out when she was 8 years old.

2. How has this impacted your child's/family's lives?

Every day in our house has challenges. We plan our trips, activities and bedtime according to what she will be able to tolerate and avoid things we know that she will just not be able to handle (known from past experiences and how she feels at that time).

3. Do you feel you have a good support system? What could improve a parent's support system?

For just over a year (age 7 - 8½ years) we had an OT who helped us through so much. It made such a difference to us all. For that time frame, we had the best support system. The parents' support we have here is wonderful. Sharing our challenges and our accomplishments has been great. We don't feel so alone through this when we get together to share our stories.

4. What has been the best advice and/or treatment you have heard or tried so far?

We have used weighted item such as blankets and weights. Another thing we have tried has been headphones, sunglasses and "just the right" brand of clothing. The biggest help, even though the earlier mentioned things have helped so much, has been picture schedules.

5. What has been the most difficult part of your child's diagnosis and what would make it easier for you?

The most difficult part has been the unknown. No two days are the same and when you think you have a handle on something, you really don't! The only thing I wish for every day for my daughter and for us as parents is continuous support. We get a few steps forward and then we "hit a wall". Therapy is short, many professionals we have dealt with don't really understand or know what she deals with every day. It feels like we are always on a lonely uphill battle.

6. How has your child's diagnosis affected them/yourself socially and emotionally?

The diagnosis is a "title" which describes how my daughter feels. It doesn't describe my daughter as the great person that she is, so it honestly hasn't affected me. One positive with it is that we now "get it" and others in our family and friends can understand when she is having a struggle or challenge.

7. Has your child's school been supportive or helpful and how? Do you have 504 plan or IEP?

The school we had been at since Kindergarten for her was horrible. They did not understand her challenges, did not "see" them and therefore did not help her at all. The trouble with SPD is that it isn't a visible disability so it is often pushed off as "nothing". We changed schools in the winter (middle of Grade 3) and the new school understands her and her needs. She is so much happier, learning so much and overall physically feels better because they help her all day long. She has what we call an IIP (Individualized Instructional Plan).

8. Has there been a positive outcome from your child's diagnosis?

The positives have been that we understand her better, family and friends understand her better and we have the ability to research and get her the help she needs.

9. What would you like the general public to know about this situation?

She is a bright, happy little girl. She wants nothing more than to do what every other kid does but is limited at times. There are times when she may not act age appropriate and that isn't because she is a bad kid or that we are bad parents. She feels, sees, smells, hears and tastes differently than we do and at times it is so bad that it hurts her. Understand...don't judge!

10. If there is anything else you would like to share with our readers on the subject, not included above, please add it here.

Dana

Macungie,USA

1. When did you first notice your child had Sensory Processing Disorder? When and how was he/she officially diagnosed?

Looking back on it, I noticed some signs when he was about 1 year old. I had never heard of SPD but my son has a speech delay and when being evaluated for that, the therapists saw signs of SPD. Over time more signs became apparent and he was officially diagnosed several weeks ago at 26 months of age.

2. How has this impacted your child's/family's lives?

I think his speech delay is related. Sleep is difficult and he either gets no naps or falls asleep very late in the day. Then there's a meltdown when we have to wake him so he will still sleep at night. Sometimes he gets up in the night and goes into my other son's room and wakes him up. We have a difficult time at gatherings - often he will meltdown with sudden surges of noise and will cling and cry for 20 minutes or more. So getting together with family and friends is difficult. We've avoided fireworks and movies because of auditory sensitivity in my older son (undiagnosed). Feeding is difficult - both my sons have foods they just refuse to eat.

3. Do you feel you have a good support system? What could improve a parent's support system?

Online support is great, but not much in "real life". Most people have never heard of SPD and don't understand it. It would be great to have specific support groups for SPD locally, maybe started by a hospital or at a community center, for parents.

4. What has been the best advice and/or treatment you have heard or tried so far?

OT is not starting until this coming Friday. I did get a weighted blanket which helps and we go to the playground often.

5. What has been the most difficult part of your child's diagnosis and what would make it easier for you?

I think the most difficult is the auditory sensitivity and needing to remove ourselves from family gatherings. I don't know what would make this easier other than to start occupational therapy.

6. How has your child's diagnosis affected them/yourself socially and emotionally?

Socially at times he is aloof and seems like he's in his own world; he just attends to one thing at a time. If he is playing with a car, he doesn't respond to someone calling his name. My son is young but at times gives tight squeezes or pushes others and I can see this affecting friendships in the future. He seems much younger than children his own age since he doesn't talk.

7. Has your child's school been supportive or helpful and how? Do you have 504 plan or IEP?

N/A - only 2 years old and not in school.

8. Has there been a positive outcome from your child's diagnosis?

At least I know what we need to do to try to help him.

9. What would you like the general public to know about this situation?

SPD is real and it doesn't mean kids are bratty or misbehaved; they simply don't handle things the same way the rest of the world does.

10. If there is anything else you would like to share with our readers on the subject, not included above, please add it here.

Sarah Chagnot

South Windsor, CT USA

1. When did you first notice your child had Sensory Processing Disorder? When and how was he/she officially diagnosed?

Her kindergarten teacher has a daughter with SPD. She noticed some of the signs right away. I noticed something was off when she blocked her ears at every little sound and hated everything.

She was diagnosed in October at the age of 5 by an OT and her developmental pediatrician.

2. How has this impacted your child's/family's lives?

We have to change a lot of the things we do with her. We have to make sure there are going to be no loud or unexpected noises and if we think there are, we have to prepare her. When it comes to other things we just try to prevent meltdowns.

3. Do you feel you have a good support system? What could improve a parent's support system?

Yes and no. People don't understand and it's frustrating, but I also have people who do understand and help.

More resources for SPD and maybe programs that can help like support groups or play groups would be an improvement.

4. What has been the best advice and/or treatment you have heard or tried so far?

Basically just listen for cues from her and the OT has helped tremendously.

5. What has been the most difficult part of your child's diagnosis and what would make it easier for you?

Trying to make her not so upset and frustrated when something happens.

6. How has your child's diagnosis affected them/yourself socially and emotionally?

She has friends that totally support her but people have also called her a baby because she gets anxious/nervous over things. Emotionally we are drained and I always think – "I don't know if I can keep doing this".

7. Has your child's school been supportive or helpful and how? Do you have 504 plan or IEP?

We are working on a 504 for her. The school has been very helpful and supportive. They are very in tune with what she needs.

8. Has there been a positive outcome from your child's diagnosis?

She has gotten a lot better with noises - with the exception of sirens, even in the distance, but a lot of other things such as bugs have improved significantly.

9. What would you like the general public to know about this situation?

Just to understand what we go through as parents on a day-to-day basis and it is not her fault the way she acts in public.

10. If there is anything else you would like to share with our readers on the subject, not included above, please add it here.

Charity Ponton

Centreville, VA, USA

1. When did you first notice your child had Sensory Processing Disorder? When and how was he/she officially diagnosed?

Sensory issues started at around 16. 18 months but he was not officially diagnosed as having SPD until 3½ when we first saw a speech pathologist and an occupational therapist for his eating issues.

2. How has this impacted your child's/family's lives?

Since he can become over stimulated easily, we have to do our outings/shopping at the quietest part of the day. Our routines have to be just so, as any change can cause a meltdown. We can't have a family vacation as he will become over stimulated because of the change in routine. I have to create two separate meals three times a day as our SPD child will only eat two things. Those are just a few of the things. Not mentioning everyday grooming, haircuts, washing hands etc. that he can't handle without crying or lashing out.

3. Do you feel you have a good support system? What could improve a parent's support system?

My husband is mostly supportive, but the extended family has been judgmental; thinking I am not disciplining, offering advice that I have repeatedly said would not work, thinking I am an over indulgent and bad parent.

There is no outside support as people do not understand SPD at all. I have one friend that has a child the same age, also with SPD, so I do at least have one person that knows what we are going through. I think the only thing that could help improve the support would be education; SPD needs to be something that people are aware of and right now there are still some medical professionals that do not recognize it as a true disability

4. What has been the best advice and/or treatment you have heard or tried

so far?

Patience and repetition. Lots of praise when our boy does something that we know is outside of his comfort zone. We are seeing an OT as well and that has also done a lot to help.

5. What has been the most difficult part of your child's diagnosis and what

would make it easier for you?

The most difficult thing is knowing that my child will probably struggle with day-to-day tasks for the rest of his life. As a mother, I am not sure there is anything that would make me not worry about that.

6. How has your child's diagnosis affected them/yourself socially

and emotionally?

I have been more depressed than I probably would be normally; I have had anxiety and stress and also had to go onto urgent care for high blood pressure which the doctor said was caused by stress. Emotionally, I worry all the time; is he getting enough to eat? Will this bath time go well? Or, will I have to hold him down again? Every day is a struggle.

7. Has your child's school been supportive or helpful and how? Do you have

504 plan or IEP?

We have received early services through our county for his speech delay but nothing in relation to the SPD. He was only recently diagnosed, so at his next IEP there may be some things added that would help to address those issues.

8. Has there been a positive outcome from your child's diagnosis?

Something positive about his diagnosis is to give me some peace of mind that it is not me doing something wrong or not doing better for my child.

9. What would you like the general public to know about this situation?

Please think before throwing judgmental looks to the mother whose child is having a meltdown in the aisle of the store. It is hard to ignore the glares and disapproving looks, especially when there is nothing that can be done that hasn't already been done.

10. If there is anything else you would like to share with our readers on the subject, not included above, please add it here.

Rachel Pigue

Panama City Beach, FL, USA

1. When did you first notice your child had Sensory Processing Disorder? When and how was he/she officially diagnosed?

At about 18 months my son stopped eating completely, he would only drink warm milk bottles. I took him to the doctor because he had always been low weight and I was freaked out that he didn't eat! He also would not sleep through the night - he cried and cried all night. The doctor started talking to me about GI issues, we ran all the biopsies and tests....nothing. He started then talking about autism because my son didn't talk either. He referred us to a neurologist, who was absolutely horrible. I had done a lot of research on my own about autism before the appointment, which took months to get into...this neurologist took one look at my son and said, "Clearly he isn't autistic because autistic children cannot show affection (as my child was hugging me) and he would be in a corner by himself." With all the research I had done, I clearly knew this was not the right information. He accused me of wanting an autism diagnosis!

After crying all the way home, I realized I had to keep fighting for answers. I found an organization in town called *Early Steps*, they come out to your home and evaluate your child, and they can offer free services up until they are 3 years old! So, they came and did the evaluation and decided he needed OT and Speech therapy. It wasn't until the OT (at Sacred Heart) had a couple of sessions with him did she start talking to me about SPD. She would have him wear special frequency headphones and do music therapy, he would learn how to finally swing, and work on his texture issues. At speech he would learn how to talk and work on his eating skills. Now my son is 2½ years old and he has improved soooo much! He still has set backs, but I'm learning that we just have to expect that. He still doesn't have the best appetite, but I think he has some oral aversions. He has in-toeing, and walks on his toes, so he now wears AFO braces. He still has trouble sleeping, wakes up about 2. 3 times a night screaming. And he still takes a bottle, mainly at night, to soothe him. He does have frequent meltdowns, and sometimes self-abuses, but we are working through it all. I feel like a diagnosis at this point doesn't matter. As long as he is getting the help he needs through therapy, then I'm thrilled! Now, when he turns 3 years old, we will start looking into further treatment if needed, and a possible diagnosis.

2. How has this impacted your child's/family's lives?

That's a loaded question! I could never express how much stress it has given me, fighting to advocate for my son. However, I'll fight for anyone I love to get what they need. The hardest part so far is still giving my daughter the same attention, and finding ways to still show her how special she is to us. Also, to explain what SPD is to my daughter and other family members is hard. Since it is a new diagnosis that is out there and it's not fully known by others, sometimes I still get the response, "There is nothing wrong with him!" I used to question myself all the time because of others' doubts. However, I realize my job is not to educate others, it's to help my son.

3. Do you feel you have a good support system? What could improve a parent's support system?

I do have a great support system! My husband is amazing, and totally there for me when I need to vent. He helps out as much as possible. My daughter is like a mini-mama, she is the sweetest big sister ever! The grandparents have been just awesome, one of whom has purchase weighted items for him because I could not financially do it. Another grandparent has been to appointments and therapy with me and has just been there for emotional support.

I think trust is very important in having a support system. Family and friends need to trust that you are only acting like a crazy lunatic because you are trying to find help!! Well, lack of sleep makes me crazy too. There are so many ways to help support someone, a simple meal delivered to your home from a friend will just make you burst into tears.

4. What has been the best advice and/or treatment you have heard or tried

so far?

Best advice I've heard has probably come from within me. I can only do what I can do, take one day at a time, expect setbacks, and treasure the moments that are amazing.

Best treatment has been those special headphones at therapy. Not noise cancelling ones, but the special frequency ones. He really seems to focus! We are trying to afford them so we can have them at home as well.

5. What has been the most difficult part of your child's diagnosis and what

would make it easier for you?

I feel like if he still needs the diagnosis at 3 years old, then that might be a battle as well. Kind of preparing myself for it. I've gotten several mixed statements about SPD, is it on the autism spectrum or isn't it? Is SPD even an official diagnosis? What would make it easier is having your child's pediatrician able to make a diagnosis! Why are we sent to specialists who see your child for 10 minutes out of one day. Makes no sense to me.

6. How has your child's diagnosis affected them/yourself socially

and emotionally?

SPD has its highs and lows. So one day he could be totally into having a play date, and the next not so sure about the new kid who is coming at him wanting to take his toys, and touch and hug him. Emotionally he does have some major meltdowns. This sometimes includes self-abuse. I have seen him bang his head on my sofa, the wall, the floor, his bed, etc. I've seen him hit himself in the face, and pull his own hair. Mostly he does this when he is frustrated, however I've seen him do it just from craving pressure. (Which is the same reason for the toe walking from what I understand.)

7. Has your child's school been supportive or helpful and how? Do you have

504 plan or IEP?

He's only 2 years old. However I've been told that, if needed, it will be a 504 plan. I have not researched that far yet.

8. Has there been a positive outcome from your child's diagnosis?

Just being able to understand a little bit into his world makes a huge difference to me. It helps me deal with meltdowns and bad days. I have also started wearing a SPD awareness bracelet (that grandma made!) and posting things on my Facebook page, just to get the word out there that there is something called SPD. Something other than autism and ADD.

9. What would you like the general public to know about this situation?

That it's real! Our world and the people in it evolve every day. So I think it's somewhat ignorant of people to say, "Well how come I've never heard of it?" or "That's the new diagnosis for ADD."

Please don't speak on issues that you know nothing about. Walk one day in my shoes, and tell me my son doesn't have sensory issues.

10. If there is anything else you would like to share with our readers on the

subject, not included above, please add it here.

Because the overall public, including many medical experts, do not have the knowledge of SPD, it will be a challenge for those of us paving the way for a new diagnosis. I'm not sure if it's curable, but I know because I advocated for my child at such a young age, that he has the best odds of living a perfectly normal life. Trust your parental instinct, I firmly believe that God put it there for a reason.

Kristie Clocksin

Mecca Indiana USA

1. When did you first notice your child had Sensory Processing Disorder? When and how was he/she officially diagnosed?

An Early Headstart teacher brought it to our attention that our son was different from other kids his age. We made a doctor's appointment, which led to an OT appointment and he was officially diagnosed a week before his first birthday.

2. How has this impacted your child's/family's lives?

His siblings don't understand and think we favor him. Other family members just don't understand and I have resorted to being a full-time stay at home mom because we cannot find child care for him.

3. Do you feel you have a good support system? What could improve a parent's support system?

We were basically in the dark when it came to SPD so we bought books and looked around the internet. We had no support system at all other than each other. I think better understanding of SPD and support groups, so you know that you are not alone, would and do help.

4. What has been the best advice and/or treatment you have heard or tried so far?

OT and Speech Therapy (ST) by far. We couldn't physically express our love for him and he couldn't do much until he started OT. Now we hug him and kiss him and are able to hold him, provided he is in the mood, and ST has helped him talk so we can understand him and his needs.

5. What has been the most difficult part of your child's diagnosis and what would make it easier for you?

The additional diagnoses along with his SPD - he has ADHD, ASD and seizures. I think better information would help.

6. How has your child's diagnosis affected them/yourself socially and emotionally?

We don't go to stores, parks or gatherings, he just cannot handle the excitement. So basically we don't get out much, he doesn't have any friends to play with other than his siblings, and I don't get any adult interaction.

7. Has your child's school been supportive or helpful and how? Do you have 504 plan or IEP?

Our school systems have actually never heard of this and we were lucky to find a special Headstart that he attends. I may have to home school him when he graduates from preschool.

8. Has there been a positive outcome from your child's diagnosis?

Yes we know what is wrong and are taking the steps to ensure he has the happiest life he could ever have.

9. What would you like the general public to know about this situation?

Better knowledge, so that when we go to the store or a restaurant we don't get stares and I don't get asked why I cannot handle my toddler's tantrums better, why is he hiding on the shelf, etc. It is not bad parenting - my child sees the world differently, that's all.

10. *If there is anything else you would like to share with our readers on the subject, not included above, please add it here.*

The best thing for me was a support group of other moms and caregivers who go through what I go through, so that I know I am not alone and if I have questions I can ask.

Laura Smith

Norman-Cleveland County

1. *When did you first notice your child had Sensory Processing Disorder? When and how was he/she officially diagnosed?*

My first indications with my son were the constant touching, jumping, spinning, and chewing. He was first diagnosed with ADHD and I had my doubts. The doctors put him on Ritalin for the ADHD and the only thing that did was make him very emotional. This is when I started doing my research and discovered Sensory Processing Disorder.

I didn't just go to his doctor and say my child has this - I documented a lot of things and also had his teachers document things that he did and what would help with keeping him focused and under control. After a year of documenting, that's when I scheduled the appointment and explained everything to the doctor. The doctor had actually never heard of SPD and was happy to know about it and how it's managed. He's been on board and the whole staff has been working very hard to get my son into OT.

2. *How has this impacted your child's/family's lives?*

SPD has actually made things easier for my family and for my child because now we are learning how to handle things and what his triggers are.

3. *Do you feel you have a good support system? What could improve a parent's support system?*

I have a wonderful support system and if anyone is unsure about something they call me. The best thing a parent can do to improve their support system is to educate them. Education is the key otherwise people just assume you have a "bad" child.

4. What has been the best advice and/or treatment you have heard or tried

so far?

The best advice and treatment is that it's ok to get overwhelmed and feel like you're doing everything wrong, but don't ever give up or blame your child or yourself and to experiment with different ways of making your child's life easier for them.

5. What has been the most difficult part of your child's diagnosis and what

would make it easier for you?

I think the most difficult part is misdiagnoses. Too many children get diagnosed with other issues or labeled as a difficult child.

6. How has your child's diagnosis affected them/yourself socially

and emotionally?

The diagnosis itself has made it easier to socialize because I know what to expect and how to change it. Emotionally nothing has really changed on my side, but I think for my child it has helped him see that it's not all his fault.

7. Has your child's school been supportive or helpful and how? Do you have

504 plan or IEP?

My child has had some amazing teachers this past school year. Prior to that he had a teacher that wasn't experienced enough to know much about disabilities in children. The teachers he has had most recently helped him learn techniques to keep him focused and were very patient with him. Yes, we have an IEP.

8. Has there been a positive outcome from your child's diagnosis?

Things couldn't be more positive now that he's been diagnosed. I'm learning what works for my child and what doesn't, as well as educating others on this disorder.

They should know that some children aren't "bad" they just have a different way of handling things.

10. If there is anything else you would like to share with our readers on the subject, not included above, please add it here.

Mary Camp

Vero Beach, FL. USA

1. When did you first notice your child had Sensory Processing Disorder? When and how was he/she officially diagnosed?

We first noticed Byron was different when he was born. His body temperature was always high. He hated certain fabrics and hated wearing pants or anything long sleeved like jackets. He was diagnosed at 2½ years of age by the OT at the therapy place we went to for his speech delay.

2. How has this impacted your child's/family's lives?

Byron has problems sitting still. He is very active so we are always trying ways to help him. It changed how we do things, and how we handle certain situations.

3. Do you feel you have a good support system? What could improve a parent's support system?

Yes, my husband, my parents and my mother-in-law have all read up on the subject. They come and visit daily and help me out a lot.

4. What has been the best advice and/or treatment you have heard or tried so far?

Best advice so far - breathe and keep breathing and use your brain. If your gut says, "Hello I'm stressing out", that's most likely what is going on with Byron. Best treatment - they used to let Byron jump into a pressure swing from high up. He loved it.

5. What has been the most difficult part of your child's diagnosis and what would make it easier for you?

6. How has your child's diagnosis affected them/yourself socially and emotionally?

Socially, I lost my sister. That hurts the most. She couldn't understand, nor would she listen, and I just couldn't take it anymore. We haven't spoken in three years. Emotionally, I used to cry and wish that Byron was normal. He has three different diagnoses: apraxia of speech, autism spectrum disorder and SPD. I still cry from time to time over it all.

7. Has your child's school been supportive or helpful and how? Do you have 504 plan or IEP?

Yes, yes and yes. Byron is attending the ESE program through our school district. He attended the autism preschool program, even though his teachers see more sensory in him then autism. Yes, he has an IEP plan and I or my husband go to every meeting.

8. Has there been a positive outcome from your child's diagnosis?

Yes, Byron has taught me so much in five years as my child. He has taught me patience, acceptance, and to enjoy my wild monkey boy. We have a 1½ year old little girl. We now look at things totally differently.

9. What would you like the general public to know about this situation?

It is not bad parenting. My son is not a spoiled brat. Sometimes he cannot control himself. It's inside of him but that doesn't stop him from being a wonderful boy. So please stop judging.

10. If there is anything else you would like to share with our readers on the subject, not included above, please add it here.

BTE Mom

Lexington, KY

1. When did you first notice your child had Sensory Processing Disorder?

When and how was he/she officially diagnosed?

I first learned about sensory processing disorder when we took our son (now 8) for an OT evaluation for a feeding disorder. He was diagnosed at that time (at age 6) and eventually my daughter was too.

2. How has this impacted your child's/family's lives?

It has made it hard to have a social life. School has been very difficult. I spend most of my time researching his disorders so it has consumed me quite a bit.

3. Do you feel you have a good support system? What could improve a

parent's support system?

I have a fair support system. I have one good friend in town who can play with my kids and understand their needs. Better support at school would help a ton.

4. What has been the best advice and/or treatment you have heard or tried

so far?

Honestly, the best advice was to have the blood test for strep. We learned he had PANDAS and a gene mutation that can be causing much of this. We plan to test our daughter next. I wish someone had suggested it years ago.

5. What has been the most difficult part of your child's diagnosis and what

would make it easier for you?

The hardest part has been convincing others that it is a real disorder, and finding answers. It would be easier for me if I had one doctor who could treat him effectively for everything.

6. How has your child's diagnosis affected them/yourself socially and emotionally?

My child is not aware of his diagnosis but he does not like social situations and it is very hard for him to make friends. I fear he will be lonely as he grows older if he doesn't learn to socialize better. I am lucky to have a set of long-time friends to lean on.

7. Has your child's school been supportive or helpful and how? Do you have 504 plan or IEP?

My son has an IEP for speech and my daughter doesn't have one at all. They score well on assessments so they don't qualify for the help they need. The school offers support in any way they can but follow through is not always good.

8. Has there been a positive outcome from your child's diagnosis?

I've met some wonderful people.

9. What would you like the general public to know about this situation?

That this is a real diagnosis and that these are not kids with slacking parents. I think awareness is very important.

10. If there is anything else you would like to share with our readers on the subject, not included above, please add it here.

I strongly believe in taking a biomedical approach to treating your child. There is no other way to know if some of their behaviors have a physical basis to them. It is not a cure, but can help your child tremendously if they have a physical reason for their sensory processing disorder.

Lora Sweeney

Bridgeton, NJ, USA

1. When did you first notice your child had Sensory Processing Disorder? When and how was he/she officially diagnosed?

I noticed right away that something was different about my son, but I didn't know why. I knew nothing about SPD and doctors told me he was just unique. One pediatrician said, "He's just at the extreme end of the Bell Curve for normal." I first learned about Sensory Processing Disorder when I took him for a Neuro/Behavioral Assessment. The psychiatrist recommended I have him evaluated by an Occupational Therapist for SPD.

He was diagnosed at 6 years old by an Occupational Therapist (December 3, 2012).

2. How has this impacted your child's/family's lives?

His special needs have had a major impact on our lives. I am currently homeschooling him because he is academically advanced, but socially, emotionally and behaviorally immature. Our regular schedule is full of appointments with Occupational Therapy, GI specialists and Behavioral Therapists. I spend a lot of time on the phone with our health insurance, billing departments, doctors and nurses. We spend quite a bit of money on copays and additional therapy/services that our insurance refuses to cover. I purchase special (and expensive) food, supplements and medications for him. We lead very structured and routine lives. We limit social engagements and outings, frequently packing him a separate meal if we are going to a place that will be serving food.

3. Do you feel you have a good support system? What could improve a parent's support system?

I have supportive family and friends, which is extremely valuable. Unfortunately, I have yet to find a supportive pediatrician or medical professional, other than Occupational Therapists. Most pediatricians and psychiatrists I have met either dismiss SPD as non-existent or have never even heard of it.

4. What has been the best advice and/or treatment you have heard or tried

so far?

The brushing has been very helpful. I hope to try listening therapy soon.

5. What has been the most difficult part of your child's diagnosis and what

would make it easier for you?

The most difficult part has been the lack of understanding from doctors and people in general. For instance, my son struggles with encopresis, partly because of Interoceptive Discrimination Disorder. However, I cannot find anyone who treats Interoceptive Discrimination Disorder or who treats encopresis from a sensory perspective.

6. How has your child's diagnosis affected them/yourself socially

and emotionally?

My son is socially and emotionally immature. It is very difficult for him to make friends. As for myself, I have actually lost one friendship because of his diagnosis.

7. Has your child's school been supportive or helpful and how? Do you have

504 plan or IEP?

My son is homeschooled. I have met resistance from the local school district in providing occupational therapy services, but I am still trying.

8. Has there been a positive outcome from your child's diagnosis?

While I am sorry for the struggles my son faces, he has developed some good strengths as well, such as persistence, determination and a huge imagination. For myself, this experience has been both humbling and enlightening. I am a stronger person and I see the world in a different way. I see both the best and the worst in people, in how they respond to my son.

9. What would you like the general public to know about this situation?

I think there needs to be more awareness of Sensory Processing Disorder.

10. If there is anything else you would like to share with our readers on the subject, not included above, please add it here.

Sonya

Davis WV

1. When did you first notice your child had Sensory Processing Disorder? When and how was he/she officially diagnosed?

I noticed and thought something was wrong from the time she was born. Diagnosis when she was aged 3 years 4 months.

2. How has this impacted your child's/family's lives?

We walk around on eggshells not knowing when the next meltdown will happen. We avoid doing things and try to think many steps ahead of time, to predict what she will do next.

3. Do you feel you have a good support system? What could improve a parent's support system?

I have a good support group with my in house family members because they have to live here and see her meltdowns. I wish that the ones who don't live here would listen when I try to tell them the ins and outs of her.

4. What has been the best advice and/or treatment you have heard or tried so far?

I am new at this but the biggest relief was receiving a diagnosis from a professional.

5. What has been the most difficult part of your child's diagnosis and what would make it easier for you?

More understanding and a local SPD parents program. Most difficult is not knowing what is wrong or what is going to happen next.

6. How has your child's diagnosis affected them/yourself socially and emotionally?

I have been able to help others with similar problems with children.

7. Has your child's school been supportive or helpful and how? Do you have 504 plan or IEP?

8. Has there been a positive outcome from your child's diagnosis?

Peace of mind, knowing that there is help.

9. What would you like the general public to know about this situation?

Just because you spend a few hours with a child doesn't mean you know them and how they are.

10. If there is anything else you would like to share with our readers on the subject, not included above, please add it here.

Don't give up.

KJB

Birmingham, AL, USA

**1. *When did you first notice your child had Sensory Processing Disorder?
When and how was he/she officially diagnosed?***

He has only been diagnosed with severe ADHD but I know he has SPD…I have known since he was quite young (5. 6 months).

2. *How has this impacted your child's/family's lives?*

We avoid things like: movie theatres (too dark and loud), riding bikes (too scary) and crowded parks (too noisy/too many people). He gets over stimulated easily and has a hard time winding down; severe insomnia also.

3. *Do you feel you have a good support system? What could improve a parent's support system?*

Not really. I have my parents and a couple of other relatives but could use a support group in the area.

4. *What has been the best advice and/or treatment you have heard or tried so far?*

Massage, compression, Epsom salt baths…letting him push heavy objects around and spin.

. *What has been the most difficult part of your child's diagnosis and what would make it easier for you?*

Knowing that he will always be just left of center.

*6. How has your child's diagnosis affected them/yourself socially
and emotionally?*

He is about 1½ years behind socially/in maturity so he tends to play with younger kids. He is very sensitive and intense emotionally.

*7. Has your child's school been supportive or helpful and how? Do you have
504 plan or IEP?*

Yes – an IEP.

8. Has there been a positive outcome from your child's diagnosis?

Yes, I know how to help him and am able to learn new things from other parents via the internet.

9. What would you like the general public to know about this situation?

That he is not a "brat" or a bad kid.

*10. If there is anything else you would like to share with our readers on the
subject, not included above, please add it here.*

Jamie Murray

Airway Heights, WA USA

1. *When did you first notice your child had Sensory Processing Disorder? When and how was he/she officially diagnosed?*

I didn't know the symptoms were SPD but, thinking back, I recall that he has had the symptoms since he was an infant. He wasn't formally diagnosed until 6 years old by a Pediatric Therapist.

2. *How has this impacted your child's/family's lives?*

It significantly impacted his developmental milestones throughout his life. In all areas: fine/gross motor, social, and behavioral skills.

3. *Do you feel you have a good support system? What could improve a parent's support system?*

I didn't have a good support system for the behavior problems. I often felt alone and no one believed me. I was a single parent most of my son's life.

4. *What has been the best advice and/or treatment you have heard or tried so far?*

Diet and Occupational Therapy geared for sensory issues, and the lycra suit has been the best treatment thus far.

5. *What has been the most difficult part of your child's diagnosis and what would make it easier for you?*

The defiance has been the most difficult part of his diagnosis. More support from family and friends.

6. How has your child's diagnosis affected them/yourself socially

and emotionally?

Due to the meltdowns and other misbehavior, we haven't been able to do things most families can do.   Church and other sit down activities have been impossible.

7. Has your child's school been supportive or helpful and how? Do you have

504 plan or IEP?

My son is homeschooled. He was evaluated by the school, but I decided to go with services out of school.

8. Has there been a positive outcome from your child's diagnosis?

He was able to get the proper treatment for best improvement in the three years since his diagnosis.

9. What would you like the general public to know about this situation?

A child that appears normal can have a behavior disability and it's not bad parenting.

10. If there is anything else you would like to share with our readers on the

subject, not included above, please add it here.

Amy Bakken

Houston, TX USA

1. *When did you first notice your child had Sensory Processing Disorder? When and how was he/she officially diagnosed?*

My son was about 6 months old when he started rocking his body incessantly. When he failed to meet many of his physical developmental milestones on time, we thought there might be a problem. He didn't sit up, crawl, stand, walk, run, talk or interact socially at the "typical" times. He never liked to show any physical affection, even though we are an extremely affectionate family. This was always a very hard thing to deal with as a mother. It feels like a bit of a rejection when your child pushes you away when you hug, kiss, embrace or even just touch them. I have to remind myself all the time that this truly isn't the case. Now, when he does show affection as he gets older it's the best thing in the world (though it is still rare). I will forever remember when he started letting me hug him and kiss him between 2 - 2½ years old. At a little over a year old, we started Early Intervention, and his therapist suggested sensory issues. I was scared to death of an autism "label" being tacked on to that. He is now almost 3 years old and making great progress, though we still struggle with sensory issues daily.

2. *How has this impacted your child's/family's lives?*

I worry that my older child will feel left out or like we are harder on her because of all the accommodations we have to make for her brother, or because of all her brother's appointments we have to take her to. I also don't want my son to feel like there is something "wrong" with him for the very same reasons.

3. *Do you feel you have a good support system? What could improve a parent's support system?*

Yes! We have been fortunate to have very supportive physicians and therapists who have taken all of our concerns very seriously. My husband is great as he is always willing to learn and try different approaches right alongside me. I hear so many other mothers (mainly only mothers) who may not have such supportive partners, or who have partners who are in denial about their child's issues. I did have one doctor (a pediatric neurologist) look at me like I was talking about voodoo when I mentioned my son had sensory sensitivities when he measured his head and my son screamed bloody murder because he is very sensitive to being touched and very apprehensive of strangers. I think one improvement would be raising awareness, even amongst the medical community, that kids DO have sensory issues without any kind of autism spectrum disorder sometimes.

4. What has been the best advice and/or treatment you have heard or tried so far?

The best advice has been "don't force it!" My son had a very strong aversion to water and so many people have told us to just put him in the tub. That would have had the opposite effect we were going for and caused so much anxiety and avoidance behaviors along with so much trauma. We literally had to start with a teaspoon full of water and work from there with such baby steps. He now walks right in the pool, and takes a bath! We are presently working on potty training with such baby steps too. Every small step and tiny bit of progress counts!

5. What has been the most difficult part of your child's diagnosis and what would make it easier for you?

Seeing the way strangers look at my child in public when he has a meltdown from being so overwhelmed or under/over stimulated. Also, people comparing my child to others. I just wish we had more people to support us without stating their own biased opinion: "He'll grow out of it." "He needs more discipline." "So and so did that too and they were fine."

6. How has your child's diagnosis affected them/yourself socially

and emotionally?

I have joined and started some moms' groups for socialization for both my child and myself and made some amazing friendships this way.

I find myself staying up till all hours of the night researching online and reading articles and books. I also have made some great connections with other mothers from internet-based groups whom I have never met in person, but have commonalities with based on our children and daily struggles and NEED for information/support.

7. Has your child's school been supportive or helpful and how? Do you have

504 plan or IEP?

We haven't reached that point yet, but I hope we don't suffer the tragic struggles I hear about!

8. Has there been a positive outcome from your child's diagnosis?

Therapy! We have made so much progress!

9. What would you like the general public to know about this situation?

These kids really cannot help it (whatever "it" is they are doing at the moment) and are learning strategies for daily living and to overcome their challenges. So are the parents! Also many adults have these issues as well!

10. If there is anything else you would like to share with our readers on the

subject, not included above, please add it here.

There is so much information out there, if you take the time to learn! There also is a great supportive community too!

Patricia

Bathurst-Australia

1. When did you first notice your child had Sensory Processing Disorder? When and how was he/she officially diagnosed?

Since my daughter was 18 months old we knew something wasn't quite right with her. She was formally diagnosed at the age of 4 by an occupational therapist.

2. How has this impacted your child's/family's lives?

It has impacted all our lives tremendously - unfortunately not in a positive way at the moment as my daughter has other diagnoses as well and is very verbal and physical, especially when having a meltdown. We have two other children and unfortunately we don't have the time we should have for them.

3. Do you feel you have a good support system? What could improve a parent's support system?

To a point I would say yes but it would be great if Sensory Processing Disorder was more recognized and more help was offered.

4. What has been the best advice and/or treatment you have heard or tried so far?

Parent and child Interactive Therapy Class.

5. What has been the most difficult part of your child's diagnosis and what would make it easier for you?

Not recognized enough and not enough understanding by the public.

6. How has your child's diagnosis affected them/yourself socially

and emotionally?

We unfortunately have lost friends and can't really go out in public as people just think we have a naughty un-disciplined child.

7. Has your child's school been supportive or helpful and how? Do you have

504 plan or IEP?

My daughter's Preschool is fantastic but I am really worried as my daughter starts Kindergarten next year and I'm worried she won't get the right support. Will be having a meeting soon for IEP.

8. Has there been a positive outcome from your child's diagnosis?

Still going through all the channels to get the right diagnoses - to make sure nothing has been missed.

9. What would you like the general public to know about this situation?

More education about Sensory Processing Disorder so that there is more understanding of it.

10. If there is anything else you would like to share with our readers on the

subject, not included above, please add it here.

Danyell Pemerton

Columbia, TN USA

1. When did you first notice your child had Sensory Processing Disorder? When and how was he/she officially diagnosed?

Looking back now I can see there were signs from when he was just an infant. I enjoyed that he preferred to lay in his crib to fall asleep rather than be rocked or that he liked to sit in a jumper instead of being held. I enjoyed my freedom.

As he grew most things were normal, he just had a few quirks - like when he crawled and had one leg come almost completely over his head, or that he didn't enjoy the same snacks as the others kids. He was still meeting all the milestones at pretty much the right times. And then around 14 months or so I had a deep down gut fear he had autism. He had so many quirks by this time like head banging, spinning, no eye contact, not sleeping, not eating and losing the words he had previously known. I was convinced he was deaf or at least had severe hearing loss because he would never respond when we talked to him. We were in the doctor's office at least twice a month for almost a whole year due to ear infections, bronchial infections, croup and even pneumonia. He did have PE tubes put in but all the hearing tests came back normal.

His doctor kept telling me everything was just fine with him and that he was on track with his height and weight so I had nothing to be concerned about. All that changed at the 18 month visit when we did the MCHAT survey. His doctor referred us for help. At this moment, six months later, we are still waiting to have a full evaluation to see the extent of what my son has going on.

I was informed about 2 months ago from one of the many evaluations we have already undergone that he has SPD. I am unsure if it is a full diagnosis as I do not know what is required to make it an actual diagnosis.

2. How has this impacted your child's/family's lives?

In a lot of ways, finding out he has SPD has made things easier. It now gives an explanation of why my son does some of the things he does. We do five hours of therapies throughout the week spread over three days and there is so much home time devoted to sensory play, stimulation and redirection. It has changed my whole outlook on my day. It seems like anything I am faced with from chores, running errands or interacting with other people I have to think about how it will affect my son now too.

I have lost contact with many people, partly because I am just so busy and partly because I don't want to over stimulate him or change a routine. It has added another obstacle in my marriage. My husband gets upset when our son goes on a quirk or with how focused on our son I have become. I have noticed my oldest son reaching out more for my attention now too. I 'm sure this is because he sees how much time I put into the younger one, I try to balance my time with them but it truly feels impossible.

3. Do you feel you have a good support system? What could improve a parent's support system?

I would love to say yes, but unfortunately I do not feel that I do. My husband and I are divided on so much. When he heard how behind our son was from the initial evaluation and there was a sensory disorder plus possibly more, he asked that I handle all of the medical issues that arose from then on. He does not want any of the actual details or diagnoses. It seems to me that most of our families either think it is "just a stage" or "all in my mind". There are a few that can see it and I can talk to, which is great, but it is one sided. It is me telling them the new thing my son is doing or how he is doing it and it is just them listening without offering advice. The very few friends I do try to maintain some contact with will listen and encourage but none have a real understanding as they have not gone through it. It honestly is only through the internet that I have any support - from online groups of other parents.

4. What has been the best advice and/or treatment you have heard or tried

so far?

The best advice came from our intake counselor. When I told her all my frustrations and challenges with the other people in our lives and all the resentment and guilt I had for myself, she told me not to give up. She told me that I am my son's main advocate, I am his voice and his understanding. It is through my love for him that I will persevere through all of this and get him functioning the best he can. Other than that therapies have been a HUGE success.

5. What has been the most difficult part of your child's diagnosis and what

would make it easier for you?

The waiting has been the hardest. Waiting to find out what his diagnoses are. Waiting on therapy to get set up. Waiting on therapy to start making a difference. Waiting for other people to understand our lives. I suppose only time will make this easier.

6. How has your child's diagnosis affected them/yourself socially

and emotionally?

I know my son loves me and others. At times I wonder if he actually knows what he is feeling and if he is capable of all the emotions I know are needed to function in society. As of now, he seems to go more off cues from others and that worries me. To be honest it has left me crying alone in the middle of night, sad about a possibility of my son's future that hopefully will never come true. I find myself emotionally drained a lot of the time.

7. Has your child's school been supportive or helpful and how? Do you have

504 plan or IEP?

My son is only 2 years old so, aside from a preschool/group therapy he will be starting, school is not an issue. We have an IEP.

8. *Has there been a positive outcome from your child's diagnosis?*

My son having sensory disorder and whatever else he may or may not have has opened up a new world for me. It has increased my awareness of others' feelings and situations. I do not plan to let my awareness end at me, I try to encourage others to broaden their awareness too.

9. *What would you like the general public to know about this situation?*

My son is normal, he is just his own normal. He cannot help what he does or the way he does it. I try very hard to help him with everything he needs, none of it is made up in my head. I am optimistic towards his future. I feel that every step we take will be in the right direction. I have faith that he will be able to rewire his brain and function "normally".

10. *If there is anything else you would like to share with our readers on the subject, not included above, please add it here.*

There are many possibilities of disorders that have similar symptoms. There needs to be much more research to be better able to tell what falls where. There are too many inconsistencies with receiving a diagnosis, one person may evaluate and say it is X while another gives the evaluation and says it is Y - there needs to be more uniformity. That will come through awareness. Also through awareness we will be able to love and care for everyone else regardless of their differences.

Candice Nichols

Kalama, USA

1. When did you first notice your child had Sensory Processing Disorder? When and how was he/she officially diagnosed?

My daughter was diagnosed with Sensory Processing Disorder when she was almost 2 years old. I had been taking her in to see a speech therapist and was discussing some of the other struggles we had been experiencing. For instance, at that time, my daughter would rock in her high chair so hard that the feet would come off the floor and the back of the chair would bang against the wall. My downstairs neighbor kept pounding on the wall whenever this happened, so I had to physically hold her high chair down every meal. After a few weeks of discussing behaviors such as this with her speech therapist, she suggested that I have my daughter evaluated for Sensory Processing Disorder. I didn't notice the early signs of SPD in my daughter because, at that time, I wasn't aware that this condition existed. Now that I am more knowledgeable about SPD, I recognize that she exhibited signs of it from infancy.

My daughter will undergo further testing next month to determine if she has any other diagnoses.

2. How has this impacted your child's/family's lives?

Sensory Processing Disorder has both positive and negative impacts on our lives. I prefer to focus on the positives.

My daughter is a combination seeker and avoider. I think that, as long as she doesn't become over stimulated by it and doesn't engage in dangerous activities, seeking sensory input can have a positive impact on her life. All of the climbing, jumping, diving, spinning, swinging, and other activities my 2½ year old engages in helps keep her healthy, fit, and happy. On the other hand, having a child who seeks vestibular input can be challenging on rainy days when we can't go to the park because she will start jumping and climbing on furniture, hitting and pinching me, jumping or climbing on me, and will have more frequent meltdowns.

My daughter seems more attuned to sights, sounds, and textures in her environment than most people, including me, and is known to suddenly stop what she is doing to investigate. For instance, we might step on a manhole cover while going for a walk and I won't even notice it, but she will suddenly stop, turn around, and stomp on it over and over again so she can hear the hollow thud it produces. If we transition from walking on grass to walking on pebbles, she will often stop to touch the different textures. For weeks, she kept doing raspberries while standing in about the same spot in my living room, but because I didn't notice the narrow shaft of light that was coming in through a slit in my blinds, I couldn't figure out why she was doing this or why she kept saying "whoa" whenever she did. Once I noticed she wasn't spitting to be naughty but was instead enthralled by watching the mist of spittle disperse and swirl through the air, I gave her a spray bottle to use instead. I think her increased awareness of sensory input helps her learn more about the world around her than she would learn if she were oblivious to these sights, sounds, and textures.

We do face a lot of struggles as a result of my daughter's sensory issues – primarily due to her avoidance of certain situations. For instance, she has had an aversion to water getting on her head since infancy. This makes washing her hair an extremely stressful task. I've tried a lot of different products and tactics in an effort to make getting her hair washed less traumatic, but so far none of them have worked.

My daughter also becomes extremely distraught in public places where there are a lot of people. I have no one to help watch her so shopping alone is not an option. This has meant that for months I have struggled to get much needed groceries.

Another challenge I face is being able to get and keep a job. My daughter goes to occupational therapy and counseling each week and I feel it is important that she continues to do this, so working a full time job is not an option. Furthermore, when I was working part time a few months ago, daycare was having problems with my daughter's behavior. Being around so many kids often left her tense and wanting to be left alone. If a child came up to her during one of these moments, she would push them and tell them "No". During the months that I worked part time, her speech development regressed and she became more violent, hitting her head against walls and the floor during meltdowns, more defiant and more apt to have a sensory-related meltdown.

3. Do you feel you have a good support system? What could improve a parent's support system?

I feel that I struggle more than a lot of parents might, due to the fact that I don't have a good support system. I'm a single mom and am raising my daughter completely alone – I do not have family, friends, or a co-parent to help. Furthermore, I am unable to access resources like respite care or Head Start because my daughter is less than 3 years old. Also, since I live in a small town, it is difficult to access some of the resources offered in cities because I struggle to afford the commute. I am aware of support groups available to parents with children who have special needs, for instance, but I simply can't afford to spend $10 in gas to go there and back.

I feel that, just as children with special needs are treated on a case-by-case basis, parents should be too. I think that for support systems to be effective they need to take into consideration what supports, if any, a parent already has and should try to fill in the gaps.

I also wish there were more resources available for families who have children with SPD who are under the age of 3.

4. What has been the best advice and/or treatment you have heard or tried so far?

Visual schedules and social stories have proven extremely effective in helping my child prepare for situations that cause her distress. It has also been helpful to teach her about emotions so she can better articulate how she is feeling. I think being able to express how she feels to me and having me respond to her emotions makes her feel more in control of the situation.

5. What has been the most difficult part of your child's diagnosis and what would make it easier for you?

The most difficult part of my child's diagnosis has been the lack of consensus on what Sensory Processing Disorder is and how to effectively treat it. There is a lot of information available for parents to access on the internet, which I eagerly consumed at a high rate right after she was diagnosed. I think it would be easier if a short and concise introduction to SPD were made available to parents upon receiving a diagnosis.

6. How has your child's diagnosis affected them/yourself socially and emotionally?

I think my child's diagnosis makes it so she is less likely to engage in social activities with other children. When she does play with other kids, they are apt to leave the vicinity if she has a meltdown, which leaves her feeling sad and disappointed.

It is really difficult to be raising a child with SPD without any friends or family. Providing extra support to my child often leaves me feeling drained.

Since my daughter struggles most in public places, the feedback I get from other parents is often in the form of looks of disapproval or pity. Due to my daughter's meltdowns and difficulties with changes in her schedule, I feel that I am further alienated from contact with other adults.

I am not typically comfortable asking for help from others, but raising a child with Sensory Processing Disorder alone has proven to be very challenging. I think that it has been good for me to become more comfortable asking for help when I need it.

7. Has your child's school been supportive or helpful and how? Do you have 504 plan or IEP?

At 2½ years old, my daughter has not yet attended school.

8. Has there been a positive outcome from your child's diagnosis?

I feel the greatest outcome from my daughter's diagnosis is that I am now aware that she has this condition and am seeking to understand it. I feel that this awareness has made it possible for me to help my child far better than I would have if I had not known she had SPD.

9. What would you like the general public to know about this situation?

I feel there is a stigma that kids who are diagnosed as having Sensory Processing Disorder are just "spoiled brats" and that their parents aren't doing their jobs. I couldn't afford to spoil my child even if I wanted to and keeping her regulated requires a lot of extra work on my part, so I am by no means a lazy or bad mom.

I would also like readers to know that the meltdown they might see my child having in the store does not define who she is. When my daughter is well-regulated, she is a sweet, polite, and helpful child. Please don't judge our children based on first impressions or un-informed biases.

10. If there is anything else you would like to share with our readers on the subject, not included above, please add it here.

1. When did you first notice your child had Sensory Processing Disorder? When and how was he/she officially diagnosed?

At 2 years old from OT, and also through other testing at 3 years old.

2. How has this impacted your child's/family's lives?

Makes things more difficult for him and for our family. Raising him is more difficult than at first.

3. Do you feel you have a good support system? What could improve a parent's support system?

No. One set of parents doesn't get it and the other set is in denial. We have few friends who we talk to about it. More education would help more to understand.

4. What has been the best advice and/or treatment you have heard or tried so far?

We are trying outpatient OT this summer. Routine and consistency has been most helpful to use.

5. What has been the most difficult part of your child's diagnosis and what would make it easier for you?

Getting his OT covered by insurance and making it closer to our home.

6. How has your child's diagnosis affected them/yourself socially and emotionally?

It has not affected him yet due to his only being 3 years old but this has taken a toll on us as parents. Since we get no breaks we are emotionally fried by the end of the day.

7. Has your child's school been supportive or helpful and how? Do you have 504 plan or IEP?

He has an IEP due to a speech delay. But they are only giving him OT through school at the lowest level available. They tell us they do not see it at school.

8. Has there been a positive outcome from your child's diagnosis?

Yes, knowing what we can do to try to help him adjust through life.

9. What would you like the general public to know about this situation?

What a day is like in the eyes of a child who has sensory processing. And also how hard and frustrating it can be on that child and the parents who raise them. EDUCATION!!!!!

10. If there is anything else you would like to share with our readers on the subject, not included above, please add it here.

Wishing there was an answer to how to help these children. Most of the time it is trial and error which in life can be frustrating and draining on all.

Sally Hoyt

Sacramento, CA U.S.A.

1. When did you first notice your child had Sensory Processing Disorder? When and how was he/she officially diagnosed?

We suspected something was going on with our child from the time he was a toddler. We didn't do anything about it until his kindergarten teacher said we should talk to our pediatrician about his low muscle tone. He was doing fine in school, but she noticed that there was "something" going on. We did an Autism screening that came up negative, but we recognized several of the characteristics from the survey in our child. We then went to an Occupational Therapist when he was 5 who did a full sensory screening and gave us the diagnosis of SPD. She described him as having low muscle tone, not knowing where his body was in space, and having a sensitivity to textures.

2. How has this impacted your child's/family's lives?

There were a lot of things we expected to do with our child, like be involved in community sports, go to community festivals, and rent bounce houses for birthday parties. We had to change our expectations as we understood the struggles our son had with those activities. We now gear our family activities to things we know he will be comfortable with like science museums, or one on one playdates. We don't go to big parties, we don't go to the county fair, and we don't often eat in restaurants because those environments are much too overwhelming for our child. Whenever we go somewhere new, we have to factor in a 20 minute transition time for him to acclimatize and be comfortable even getting out of the car.

3. Do you feel you have a good support system? What could improve a parent's support system?

Luckily we have a great support system of family and friends who understand and make allowances for our son. What helped it become this way is the discussions I had with them about what is going on with our son and why. For example, once they understood why he shied away from giving hugs, they were much more accepting of just asking him for a high-five instead.

4. What has been the best advice and/or treatment you have heard or tried so far?

The best advice I have been given is to find things that make him happy and pursue those activities. I shouldn't make him do something like ride his bike just because society expects it. Instead, it's OK if he runs beside the other kids who are on their bikes.

5. What has been the most difficult part of your child's diagnosis and what would make it easier for you?

The most difficult part of the diagnosis was actually seeing it on paper. When I got the report back and saw that he truly was struggling in many areas of his life, it was heartbreaking. After I got over that, the report became a tool that truly helped me understand him.

6. How has your child's diagnosis affected them/yourself socially and emotionally?

The diagnosis has affected my 8 year old son in many ways. It takes him a long time to make friends. He prefers to play by himself, and knows he is different to most kids in this way. He is fearful of playground equipment, and he knows that other kids are not. He has never asked for a friend to come over and play. He does not like to leave the house. If we go on vacation, he prefers to stay in the hotel, or at least come back to the hotel in between activities. He is a happy kid when he is in his comfort zone, but take him out of it and it is really stressful for both him and me. For myself, I am a very social person who likes to be on the go. I have had to limit my activities to match his comfort level. To counter this, I make sure to go out when my husband gets home, or have my family watch him while I go shopping.

We do not have a 504 or an IEP because SPD is not a recognized disability. So far, I have not had a need to push for any accommodations because he does fine academically. He is going into 3rd grade next year, and each year I have made sure to communicate with his teacher about struggles he might have like taking longer to write, or needing a comfortable place to transition from a chaotic activity. Because I am a teacher myself, it has been easy for me to form a relationship with his teachers. I try to come into the classroom as much as possible so I can see how he is interacting and how he functions in the classroom.

I have needed more support from the cafeteria and playground staff because that is where he really struggles. The cafeteria is too bright, loud, and smelly for him to be comfortable, so he often doesn't eat much lunch. The playground is very unstructured and physical, so he prefers to run the line that separates the grass from the blacktop by himself. I made sure to talk to the supervisory staff to let them know why he does this so they don't try to force him into anything. They also know that if he gets hurt that he needs a quiet place by himself with no one touching him and he will calm down. They have been very supportive once they understand why he reacts the way he does.

8. Has there been a positive outcome from your child's diagnosis?

The most positive outcome is that we understand him better. Once we knew why he only liked soft clothes, it was easier to accommodate him. Once we knew that he tires faster than expected because he has low muscle tone, we could plan ahead for how much activity we allowed. The more we learn about SPD, the better we are able to help him negotiate the world.

9. What would you like the general public to know about this situation?

I want people to understand that all children are unique and to look beyond behaviors before judging the child.

Kirstie Steptoe

Princes Risborough, Bucks United Kingdom

1. When did you first notice your child had Sensory Processing Disorder? When and how was he/she officially diagnosed?

My daughter was different to her older brothers from an early age. She was only diagnosed in June 2013 by her pediatrician who saw her several times.

2. How has this impacted your child's/family's lives?

She is hard work and constantly on the go. I feel sorry for my older boys as they do miss out on a lot of things.

3. Do you feel you have a good support system? What could improve a parent's support system?

I don't have much support apart from the group on Facebook. An improvement would be if Sensory Processing Disorder was more commonly known in the United Kingdom.

4. What has been the best advice and/or treatment you have heard or tried so far?

We are still in the early days.

5. What has been the most difficult part of your child's diagnosis and what would make it easier for you?

More information for parents and siblings.

6. How has your child's diagnosis affected them/yourself socially

and emotionally?

My daughter only has a limited number of friends she plays with. She likes to play alone.

7. Has your child's school been supportive or helpful and how? Do you have

504 plan or IEP?

My daughter's school has been excellent and very understanding along the way, we have an IEP.

8. Has there been a positive outcome from your child's diagnosis?

Yeah there has - my daughter is no longer being called a naughty child by other kids.

9. What would you like the general public to know about this situation?

It shouldn't be a taboo subject. I think that it should be a well-known disorder in the world.

10. If there is anything else you would like to share with our readers on the

subject, not included above, please add it here.

Ingrid Fehr

Waterlooville, England

1. When did you first notice your child had Sensory Processing Disorder? When and how was he/she officially diagnosed?

We noticed that our daughter was different from a very young age. When she was less than 2 years old she had some two piece puzzles (numbers, letters and opposites) and she would put them together in the same order every time. In fact, if we tried to do it in a different order she would get very upset.

We took her to several specialists but no one was ever any help in determining a diagnosis. It wasn't until she started school at age 4 that people started taking it more seriously as she was having so many behavioral issues. We finally got to see CHAMS (Child Health and Mental Services) and the first person we saw was unfortunately no help at all. She observed our daughter and did not seem to have any ideas. We saw another person and she said SPD. She told us to get *The Out of Sync Child* and it was as if someone wrote a book about our daughter, we could see so many of her behaviors in the book!!

2. How has this impacted your child's/family's lives?

Knowing what we are dealing with has made all the difference in the world! I used to say to my daughter "look at me when I am talking to you!" and now I know that she can't. We used to wonder why she screamed when she saw fireworks, or couldn't sit in a movie theatre without clamping her hands on her ears.

While we do still have lots of issues, it makes all the difference in the world to know there is a reason for it. Before the diagnosis we doubted ourselves as parents and wondered if it was us. We have also received support which has made a great deal of difference too. At one point I almost lost my job as she was sent home from school so often. My husband and I also almost split due to the stress of everything that was happening. We are a much stronger family now as we have a better idea of how to cope with things. It is still hard (REALLY hard on some days). A diagnosis does not make issues go away, but it makes a world of difference.

3. Do you feel you have a good support system? What could improve a parent's support system?

Yes and no. I don't think there is enough understanding about SPD which makes it hard. Also as it is not a fully agreed upon disability you do not get the same support that you would for something like autism. The school that my daughter is at has been wonderful but the first school she was at didn't want to deal with it. They kept saying "other kids do not cause us any issues".

We do not have any other family here so when anything happens we have to leave work which has caused us significant issues.

Another problem is just finding the different support that may be available. If you do not know what is out there, how do you find it?

4. What has been the best advice and/or treatment you have heard or tried so far?

One thing that has really helped has been getting her a chew necklace (chewigem). Previously she was chewing her fingers to the point that they would bleed. She now has a necklace that she wears everywhere she goes and her fingers are healing well. She still chews her nails but at least her fingers are ok.

5. What has been the most difficult part of your child's diagnosis and what would make it easier for you?

The worry about how she will cope as she gets older. She struggles making friends and it is so hard when you see that she does not have anyone that she is particularly close to. I also worry how this will be as she gets older and tries to find a job. How will she handle her meltdowns, etc. Now she is young and while most people don't understand her meltdowns there is still a bit more understanding. Once she is an adult there will be no compassion for any behavior issues and how will she cope?

6. How has your child's diagnosis affected them/yourself socially and emotionally?

Is has certainly helped her as at school the staff is much more understanding of her issues. They can see when she is on edge and can help her to calm down before a full meltdown. It is the same at her after school/holiday club. CHAMS did some training sessions with the staff which they have said have helped with our daughter as well as other students.

It is hard for parents of other kids. She has hurt other children and they do not understand her condition. We do not try to force anything on anyone but as most people have never heard of SPD I think some people think you are making it up as an excuse.

Her diagnosis has helped us though as we are still a complete family. As I previously mentioned we were close to splitting due to the stress of her behavior. The diagnosis has allowed us to take some of the pressure off ourselves as we no longer blame ourselves for her struggles. It has also allowed us to recognize the same sorts of behavior in family members (my sister and my husband's brother). It does make us wonder if they would have struggled less if this was recognized in the past.

7. Has your child's school been supportive or helpful and how? Do you have 504 plan or IEP?

My daughter's current school has been extremely supportive, however her first school was not at all. My daughter has a statement which has allowed them some additional support which has proved very successful. They also have a nurture group at the school which allows my daughter and some of the other students to have additional support. Through this my daughter has made great improvements in her behavior.

8. Has there been a positive outcome from your child's diagnosis?

Yes, this allows us, her teachers and after school/holiday club staff to better understand why she behaves the way she does. People are much more patient and understanding when they realize that there is a reason she behaves the way she does.

9. What would you like the general public to know about this situation?

I think it is extremely important for the general public to become aware of SPD and that it is a genuine diagnosis. Almost everyone knows what autism and ADHD is but I have never met anyone that knows what SPD is and how it affects those with it.

It is so hard if you are out in public and your child has a meltdown. Most children with SPD look completely "normal" and so people simply think they are badly behaved. When this happens and people look at you and your child like you are bad parents and your child is just a spoiled brat, it makes you and your child feel awful. My daughter doesn't understand when people look at her and talk about her and it makes her feel awful and in her words "stupid".

10. If there is anything else you would like to share with our readers on the subject, not included above, please add it here.

I just want people to take a bit of time and learn about SPD and how it affects people. Try to imagine what it is like when your senses completely bombard you and do not allow you to concentrate on anything. Try to imagine not being able to listen to someone talking to you while looking at them as when you look at them you are completely distracted by their facial expressions. That when there are loud noises it feels ten times louder to you to the point that you are in physical pain. If you do not suffer with this you can never understand what they are going through and the constant battle that daily life can be. People with SPD are just trying to cope and survive and they need society to accept and understand them.

Naomi Mae Conto

Lucas, U.S.A

1. When did you first notice your child had Sensory Processing Disorder? When and how was he/she officially diagnosed?

When our son was 18 months old he started lining up all his toys that he played with, and when he was 24 months old he was putting together 24 piece puzzles with no help. He is currently almost 6 and does 100-piece puzzles. He hasn't been diagnosed as of yet. We have an appointment to get that in December along with being assessed for Asperger's Syndrome.

2. How has this impacted your child's/family's lives?

He has a lot of trouble with loud noises, sunlight, wearing clothes, expressing emotions, has many meltdowns, doesn't sit still, always on the go .. moving.

3. Do you feel you have a good support system? What could improve a parent's support system?

No and yes, I have a few friends that listen to me and lend me an ear but they don't live in the same state as me. Other than my husband no one helps me out or lends me support in any way, they feel there is nothing wrong with him.

4. What has been the best advice and/or treatment you have heard or tried so far?

Weighted blankets to help calm him down and with the help of Melatonin let him sleep through the night.

5. What has been the most difficult part of your child's diagnosis and what would make it easier for you?

The cost of weighted blankets and other sensory help device are hard to obtain and pay for.

6. How has your child's diagnosis affected them/yourself socially and emotionally?

He tends to play by himself or with just one or two other children.

7. Has your child's school been supportive or helpful and how? Do you have 504 plan or IEP?

This year he will be in Kindergarten, he already has an OT and will have a speech therapist and will qualify for IEP. Last year in preschool, he had a teacher that had been trained to deal with children with issues such as my son has.

8. Has there been a positive outcome from your child's diagnosis?

As stated above he hasn't been diagnosed yet, but I am hoping that it leads to more understanding and awareness.

9. What would you like the general public to know about this situation?

That it is a real medical issue, and to be more understanding about health problems that can't physically be seen.

10. If there is anything else you would like to share with our readers on the subject, not included above, please add it here.

Although the job of being a parent to a child with SPD is tiring and demanding, I have to say I wouldn't change my son or want him any other way than he is. He has his up and downs, his good days and his bad days. Just like it is with any other child.

Alexandria Glare

Westminster, CA USA

1. When did you first notice your child had Sensory Processing Disorder? When and how was he/she officially diagnosed?

I first noticed when he was about 3 years old, but his doctors felt that it was in relation to chemotherapy treatments and would "go away" over time. When it didn't go away, we brought it up again, and his pediatrician reviewed everything and told us she thought he had SPD and wanted to send him for evaluations. Evaluations showed that he likely has SPD, and that while it's possible it is a result of treatment, it is also possible that it's not.

2. How has this impacted your child's/family's lives?

We have to plan things better. Before, we would do a lot of spontaneous trips and activities. Now we need time to prepare him. When we do have something spontaneous, we have to be prepared for meltdowns. We also found that he is absolutely terrified of social situations, and if prepared he does OK, but if not prepared he will have a meltdown.

3. Do you feel you have a good support system? What could improve a parent's support system?

In some ways yes. My mom has been wonderful and my husband is trying to be. But I think if the doctors had not marked it off for so long, we would have had a lot more support from friends.

4. What has been the best advice and/or treatment you have heard or tried so far?

This is all very new to us, but the best advice we have gotten so far is to actively seek an IEP for him and request supportive therapies.

5. What has been the most difficult part of your child's diagnosis and what would make it easier for you?

The unknown. We are still at the stage where we are figuring it out, and learning to adapt around my son's needs.

6. How has your child's diagnosis affected them/yourself socially and emotionally?

He doesn't know he has SPD. He's only 5 years old. But I see him want to be with other kids, but afraid to at the same time. For me, it has been a relief. Because I can finally understand more and I no longer feel like I am somehow failing him.

7. Has your child's school been supportive or helpful and how? Do you have 504 plan or IEP?

My son is just starting Kindergarten and we are requesting an IEP. I spoke with the special education director of our charter school and she seems to be very on board.

8. Has there been a positive outcome from your child's diagnosis?

Yes, he is starting to get help because we are starting to understand his needs and be able to work with and through them.

9. What would you like the general public to know about this situation?

Don't look at a parent whose child is different from what you consider normal and judge them to be bad parents, and don't judge our children as out of control. We are doing the best we can with limited information and trying to help our children to learn to live in YOUR world when you can't or won't meet them in theirs. Sometimes that means wearing earmuffs at the beach in 100 degree weather, and that's OK. Because it means they are adapting to YOUR world.

10. *If there is anything else you would like to share with our readers on the subject, not included above, please add it here.*

Even though we accept our children for who and what they are, we can still grieve the loss of normalcy in our lives. We are not saying we don't love our children. We're saying that we didn't expect it to be so difficult to help our children live in the world you live in. Our children have different ways of living in this world. Sometimes they need quiet, sometimes they need movement, and sometimes they just need understanding. They aren't "bad kids" any more than I am a "bad mom", they are simply unique.

Jillian Hill

Saint Clair, United States

1. When did you first notice your child had Sensory Processing Disorder? When and how was he/she officially diagnosed?

He has always been different. I noticed when he was a baby. I tried breastfeeding him and he never got enough. I was so sore because he would feed for hours. Then we didn't know he had a double ear infection or that he was teething until I took him for his 6 months doctor visit. His gums were bruised but the pain didn't faze him. Finally he was in kindergarten and his teacher had been an OT before she became a kindergarten teacher. She had the school's OT come and she did some tests. His pediatrician agreed with the diagnosis. He will be going to regular OT sessions starting next month.

2. How has this impacted your child's/family's lives?

The biggest issue is his eating habits. He will not tolerate certain foods. Picky doesn't even come close to describing what he will or won't eat. I usually end up making two different meals so I know he gets something to eat as well. He has recently started trying things he normally wouldn't. If he gets off his daily routine he has been known to have complete meltdowns or have trouble sleeping because of his anxiety.

3. Do you feel you have a good support system? What could improve a parent's support system?

I wish I could say I had a great support system. My husband is doing better with helping with our son and his parents recently started trying to help but I don't really have anybody else in my life. I am currently a stay at home mom and it's really hard because I sometimes feel forgotten by the rest of the world. Thing would be better if my family tried to be in the picture or even just called sometimes. Or if any of the people that are supposed to be my friends would pick up a phone once in a while. His school is great with him though.

4. What have been the best advice and/or treatment you have heard or tried

so far?

The best thing we have is sticking with a routine as much as possible. Also if there is a deviation to the normal schedule makes sure he has enough notice so he can cope better. Giving him baths in lavender Epson salt keeps him more relaxed at bed time. I also give him a massage before bed with lavender bedtime lotion. He seems to sleep better if we stick with doing these things before bedtime. He loves tight hugs and when he is having a meltdown sometime that helps him come back from it.

5. What has been the most difficult part of your child's diagnosis and what

would make it easier for you?

Honestly just knowing that there is a name for it has made our lives easier because we know there is help with out there and he will be ok. The meltdowns are the most stressful times because he just isn't himself when they happen. Knowing a little bit more about what to do for him would make things easier but we are working on that.

6. How has your child's diagnosis affected them/yourself socially

and emotionally?

It hasn't affected anything about his life. He is just another kid to his peers and that's the way we hope it stays. If anything, his quirks have made him more popular than we ever thought was possible. We can't go anywhere in our town without someone from his class or school going out of their way to be noticed by him.

7. Has your child's school been supportive or helpful and how? Do you have

504 plan or IEP?

They have been very helpful with him. He wasn't getting what he needed from his first teacher so they moved him for us to another class (with the teacher I mentioned earlier) and it's been downhill ever since. He doesn't have a 504 plan or IEP yet so far but school starts up again next week so we will see if that changes.

8. Has there been a positive outcome from your child's diagnosis?

We handle things better with him because we try to read up on how to work with him. The most positive thing is, as I said before, he is going to be ok.

9. What would you like the general public to know about this situation?

If you see a child screaming or throwing a tantrum in public it's not always because they are spoiled or not disciplined enough - sometimes it's because they are going through something. Staring and acting like their parents are horrible people because their kid is freaking out doesn't help. Sometimes a little understanding would be great. Don't always assume you know what's going on.

10. If there is anything else you would like to share with our readers on the subject, not included above, please add it here.

I know I am my son's biggest advocate. I am here to protect and support my child through the journey he has been forced to take. Don't let you child feel alone in this because they are special and if they can't count on you who can they count on? It's going to be hard at times and you are going to want to pull your hair out. You are going to go through rough patches yourself but I don't know of anything that is more worth my time than my children.

Kelli Flores

Atwater, CA USA

1. When did you first notice your child had Sensory Processing Disorder?

When and how was he/she officially diagnosed?

I started noticing my daughter, who is a twin, having sensory issues around age 2. I had her diagnosed through the school district as a learning problem rather than as a medical problem in fear of consequences if she wanted to get a federal job, so she was diagnosed with autistic-like behaviors/SPD. She was 4 when we had her evaluated.

2. How has this impacted your child's/family's lives?

Understanding why she acts out or goes into meltdowns has made a difference in how we deal with her. We know to avoid certain situations as they may "trigger" her into a meltdown. After having her evaluated for SPD/ASD she has started a new school to help teach her coping skills, and how to handle certain stimuli and find a space where she can decompress and refocus.

3. Do you feel you have a good support system? What could improve a

parent's support system?

Yes, I feel through the SPD Facebook website I am NOT ALONE!! Big support hearing from other parents going through similar situations, I have gleaned a lot of good information from the site. Her school is very supportive and they have a good line of communication between staff and parents. Since she started at the beginning of May she has made good improvement. She will continue to go to the school until Kindergarten then will mainstream out into public schools possibly doing Resource if she needs extra support.

4. What has been the best advice and/or treatment you have heard or tried so far?

There has been a lot of advice, I think helping her with her "seeking" behavior like getting trampolines for her to use, or using ear muffs to help her avoid sounds that make her upset. Learning how to deal with meltdowns, the triggers and how to redirect has been helpful from other parents and staff at her school.

5. What has been the most difficult part of your child's diagnosis and what would make it easier for you?

I believe I was in denial about her behaviors, and getting the diagnosis through the evaluation was heartbreaking yet a relief. We finally got the answer we knew we were going to get but we also received the support needed to help her out. I don't believe there is any "easy" way of having your child diagnosed, it's very personal and very hard to have to admit that your child may have special needs. I think as long as you have a good rapport with those whom are evaluating your child and they allow you to have your input and incorporate that into the therapy, then that makes it easier for everyone; especially the child.

6. How has your child's diagnosis affected them/yourself socially and emotionally?

There is no difference. We have genetic traits that come from my mother's side and my husband's side of the family that show our kids were bound to get one of those traits. I think knowing what triggers her makes it easier to let others know when she is about to have a meltdown. I can explain that she's not just being a "brat" but has a disorder that interferes with her ability to process information.

7. Has your child's school been supportive or helpful and how? Do you have

504 plan or IEP?

My daughter goes to a specialized school and they are AWESOME!!! I wish they could live with us!!! We have an IEP for our daughter.

8. Has there been a positive outcome from your child's diagnosis?

Knowledge is power! Finally getting my head out of the sand and having her evaluated was the best positive outcome. We now have a foundation on how to help her cope with her disorder and hope that she will be able to move forward in the future, possibly not having to have specialized therapy.

9. What would you like the general public to know about this situation?

I would like them to know that children with SPD are not "brats" they are not acting out because they want to but because they simply do not know how to cope with the overwhelming amount of stimuli coming at them. SPD is not something you just outgrow, or can "beat" out of them! It is who they are and how they interpret the world around them. If more people understood what SPD is they may find out that they themselves might have a few indicators of SPD.

10. If there is anything else you would like to share with our readers on the

subject, not included above, please add it here.

We have become a world of technology, we are inundated with information much faster than 40 years ago when I was a child. Looking at some of the games, baby toys, television shows for children and video games it's no wonder that our kids are overwhelmed; as an adult I am overwhelmed trying to process information myself! I think we need to re-evaluate all the stimuli out there and perhaps tone it down a bit, infants and toddlers are exposed to too much information for their young minds to handle.

Sandy M Palmer

Orlando, FL / USA

1. When did you first notice your child had Sensory Processing Disorder? When and how was he/she officially diagnosed?

2 to 3 weeks after birth - I couldn't dress her without her screaming. No official diagnosis but OT, PT, Peds and Neuro all said the same thing.

2. How has this impacted your child's/family's lives?

HUGE impact. You learn to live around the meltdowns by rehearsing settings and making sure to ease the child into things instead of just doing them.

3. Do you feel you have a good support system? What could improve a parent's support system?

Not really but I have learned to manage. My husband works out of Afghanistan and my family thinks conditions are only an excuse for bad behavior.

4. What has been the best advice and/or treatment you have heard or tried so far?

Brush therapy and exposure over and over. Time / age.

5. What has been the most difficult part of your child's diagnosis and what would make it easier for you?

More help. More people, especially schools, being educated. Helmet therapy for plagiocephaly and PT for torticollis were some of the hardest to deal with. Lots of crying.

*6. How has your child's diagnosis affected them/yourself socially
and emotionally?*

Haven't stopped fighting the system. Socially we tend to find families with similar children so it's really not too big of a deal. We do have issues with other kids not understanding and bullying my daughter.

*7. Has your child's school been supportive or helpful and how? Do you have
504 plan or IEP?*

We had a 504 but only because I ended up testing privately and threatening with attorneys. School fought me every step of the way. We have a McKay Scholarship now and took her out of that school. Starting private this year and they are aware of her processing difficulties.

8. Has there been a positive outcome from your child's diagnosis?

Yes, that I understand why she does things. She is the sweetest girl.

9. What would you like the general public to know about this situation?

So they don't keep making uneducated ignorant statements about these wonderful children who do not have bad behavior but that aren't able to express themselves like regular children do.

*10. If there is anything else you would like to share with our readers on the
subject, not included above, please add it here.*

These children are so much more in tune with things and they will pick up on your body language without you ever knowing they did, so to try and fake friendly will not work. Be aware of how you act and what you say.

Dorinda Richardson

Everett, USA

1. When did you first notice your child had Sensory Processing Disorder? When and how was he/she officially diagnosed?

I had always known there was something different about him, but until he was diagnosed with SPD I honestly didn't know. He had some assessments done last year around November and December. He will be going through further testing for other additional conditions soon, hopefully.

2. How has this impacted your child's/family's lives?

It is a constant awareness and education factor for me to explain to friends and family about his condition. I am much busier with appointments now that he is in OT Therapy.

3. Do you feel you have a good support system? What could improve a parent's support system?

When he was first diagnosed I was at a complete loss, not really knowing anything about the condition. Since then I have become very active with an online support group that tries to arrange events to go to together. I believe the main thing is spreading awareness as much as possible so children can be diagnosed earlier and parents may start to see traits sooner than later.

4. What has been the best advice and/or treatment you have heard or tried so far?

We recently were able to acquire a weighted blanket which my son loves and it helps him to fall asleep much faster at naptime at daycare and at bedtime at home.

5. What has been the most difficult part of your child's diagnosis and what
would make it easier for you?

I believe trying to remember the difference between him acting out and having an actual meltdown. I think just trying different techniques of calming and trying to recognize the triggers before it happens helps.

6. How has your child's diagnosis affected them/yourself socially
and emotionally?

I'm not sure that he understands his condition exactly. I became very anti-social after getting the diagnosis until I started to research more. Once I learned more about ways to help him I felt more comfortable taking him places. For the most part he's always been a social child so that didn't really change. He's also always been very sensitive so emotionally I didn't really see a change in him either.

7. Has your child's school been supportive or helpful and how? Do you have
504 plan or IEP?

My son isn't school age yet. He started Head Start at his daycare a few weeks ago. His daycare's child specialist and on site doctor are the ones who originally assessed him in the classroom and gave me information on getting further testing and then therapy. We have definitely worked as a team to try to keep everyone on the same page with him. It has been somewhat difficult to figure out what works with him and what doesn't since something that works at home one on one may not work in class with 19 other children. Currently we have not created a 504 plan or IEP yet.

8. Has there been a positive outcome from your child's diagnosis?

It was just nice to find out that it wasn't something I did or didn't that made him the way he is. I have been making as many people aware of his condition including family and friends. I think it has brought my family closer together now that they know he's not normally acting out, he's actually over stimulated and having a meltdown.

9. *What would you like the general public to know about this situation?*

I just want people to know that there is help and support out there. You are not alone and until my son was diagnosed I didn't know just how common the condition has become. It seems I have several friends that have children with similar or same conditions that I've been able to help further through my awareness and the resources I tell people about.

10. *If there is anything else you would like to share with our readers on the subject, not included above, please add it here.*

N/A

Sarah Heard

Heber Springs, United States

1. When did you first notice your child had Sensory Processing Disorder?

When and how was he/she officially diagnosed?

My daughter was 16 months old when I suspected she might be autistic or semi-autistic. I told her father and he blew it off, saying she was just a bad child and needed more discipline. Of course, that didn't change things. She got worse and worse. At the age of 4, we moved to another location away from her father, and she began school the next fall. She had discipline problems in school, had difficulty sitting still, so the Kindergarten Teacher and school counselor asked if they could do an evaluation for ADHD. Not only did she have ADHD, but she had SPD as well.

2. How has this impacted your child's/family's lives?

People look at us as if we are bad parents because our child is so out of control (according to most in society).

3. Do you feel you have a good support system? What could improve a

parent's support system?

I have an excellent support system including my husband (my daughter's step-father), my parents and online groups.

4. What has been the best advice and/or treatment you have heard or tried

so far?

Occupational Therapy and using headphones in noisy situations helps a lot.

5. What has been the most difficult part of your child's diagnosis and what

would make it easier for you?

At first it was trying to understand WHY this was part of her life, and learning how to help her. It was frustrating at first because I didn't know what to do, or how to help her.

6. How has your child's diagnosis affected them/yourself socially and emotionally?

It hasn't really affected our social life. Emotionally, it's difficult every single day. Every day is a challenge and struggle for all of us. She wants to be like the other kids, and cries about it. "Why can't I just be like all the other kids at school, mama?" I have cried with her through the good times, and the bad.

7. Has your child's school been supportive or helpful and how? Do you have 504 plan or IEP?

Yes, she has an IEP plan. She does some school work at school but most of her school work is sent home to work on one on one with mama. She doesn't have as heavy a load of school work as the other kids, because she simply can't handle it. The school is understanding. She also goes to OT through the school three times a week.

8. Has there been a positive outcome from your child's diagnosis?

Yes, it helped me understand what was wrong with her, and how to better help her cope with problems that we had, in the past, thought were discipline issues.

9. What would you like the general public to know about this situation?

Our children are wonderful blessings, little people full of life, with loving hearts. They have fun personalities that make them wonderful people. Yes, they have issues. Yes, to some they may look like they are hateful little people, but in honesty they are not. They have issues, and problems just like the rest of us. They want to be accepted and loved for who they are, not what the world wants them to be!

Shandi M. Foster

Thomasville, NC USA

1. When did you first notice your child had Sensory Processing Disorder? When and how was he/she officially diagnosed?

I knew something was not quite right from birth. My son didn't want to be held, didn't want to be swaddled, and was quite sensitive to touch, sound, breast milk, formulas, etc. I mentioned SPD and autism to our pediatricians for several years and they said he was normal (because that's easily assessed by spending 10 minutes with him…right). Finally, when he was 5 years old and entering Pre-K, I spoke with his favorite pediatrician and she pre-diagnosed him with SPD but marked it as delayed development due to his fine motor skill issues (as SPD is not a recognized medical diagnosis) and referred us to an awesome Occupational Therapist who finalized the diagnosis. He will be entering Kindergarten in a few weeks and we are very pleased with his progress!

2. How has this impacted your child's/family's lives?

SPD, before we knew for sure of his diagnosis, was complete chaos for our family if I'm to be completely honest. I love my son with all of my heart and it felt so defeating not knowing how to help him or what he was feeling and needing during his challenging moments. Now that we've got his diagnosis and been working with the pediatrician and his OT, as well as the educational system in our city, my husband and I feel much more equipped to help him get through obstacles. And because of the literature available now and the Sensory Processing Disorder parent support group page on Facebook I am much more educated on the subject and can easily explain it to others. There are so many parents that understand just what I'm dealing with and give great advice!

3. Do you feel you have a good support system? What could improve a

parent's support system?

I have a great support system through the support group page on Facebook, my son's pediatrician and occupational therapist as well as through the school system. My family, however, is quite traditional and are still skeptical about his diagnosis and, similarly to many other people, like to make judgments about bad parenting. My other child doesn't have SPD and has no issues in behavior so logically this isn't so.

I think the best way to improve a parent's support system is to educate the general public with SPD awareness. The educational system is learning more about SPD every day but we also need to spread awareness to the community and let them know that this is real and these children and their families need their support to improve these children's progress.

4. What has been the best advice and/or treatment you have heard or tried

so far?

The best treatments for my son's specific issues were the brushing therapy, weighted pillows, blankets, vests, and fine motor manipulation therapy with ball barons and silly putty. Behaviorally we learned things that trigger certain meltdowns and have slowly introduced him to those triggers to allow him to acclimatize himself to his environment and have made vast improvements with his sensitivities to light, sound, and certain textures. He can now calm himself the majority of the time and even brushes himself when he feels he needs it.

5. What has been the most difficult part of your child's diagnosis and what

would make it easier for you?

The most difficult part of my son's diagnosis was getting the medical community to recognize it as an issue. Resources for these types of diagnoses are not in abundance in the area we live in so it was very difficult to get a diagnosis at all. The medical community and OT community need to work together and do more extensive research on SPD to help families have more resources.

6. How has your child's diagnosis affected them/yourself socially and emotionally?

My son is very sensitive and can be quite aggressive socially so he has meltdowns a lot in large groups of kids (improving of course) and this causes others to avoid him sometimes. He loves people and loves to play with other kids. He yearns for human contact so much but sometimes it overwhelms him and his feelings get hurt. It is emotionally disheartening for all of us because I want nothing more than for him to be happy and it hurts my heart to see him go through these obstacles because of his SPD.

It was very emotionally traumatizing for my husband and I before the diagnosis because he would literally cry all the time and never sleep. We couldn't comfort him the way he needed and we felt helpless…I'm sure my son did too.

7. Has your child's school been supportive or helpful and how? Do you have 504 plan or IEP?

The school systems have been supportive so far. They have suggested that he stay in regular class rooms and they would assess his need for exceptional class if needed. We do not have a 504 plan but the school did mention assessment of an IEP. At his Kindergarten assessment they stated that the IEP would most likely not be needed as he seems to have progressed well.

8. Has there been a positive outcome from your child's diagnosis?

I thank God every day that we got his diagnosis because now we know how to handle it and how to treat it. We can help our son and we can also help others who felt helpless like we did. WE ARE NOT ALONE! My son is the positive outcome. I have seen him feel defeated by his sensory issues and now I watch him progress daily – he brushes his teeth now with no problems, he can get wet now without having a meltdown, he can reason with himself and others when he is having sensory overload, he is reading and writing and doing so many things that we were once convinced he would either never do or take so long to accomplish. He is my miracle and a true inspiration to me every day!

9. What would you like the general public to know about this situation?

SPD parents and children are fighting a battle, some small and some large. Please if you see a parent or child having a hard time with something, offer a consoling smile. Don't label these parents as "bad parents" (they already ask that of themselves enough) and don't label these dear children as "bad behavior kids". We need to lift these kids up and give them a positive view of themselves, we should not condemn them to a negative self-fulfilling prophecy.

Be understanding and open-minded when you hear that someone has been diagnosed with SPD. Educate yourselves about SPD in order to help others.

10. If there is anything else you would like to share with our readers on the subject, not included above, please add it here.

Mary Kemper

Greenville South Carolina, USA

1. When did you first notice your child had Sensory Processing Disorder? When and how was he/she officially diagnosed?

Last fall we went on a Caribbean vacation. My little guy (18 months at the time) sat in the stroller the entire week because he absolutely could not stand to have his feet in the sand. At the time we didn't think much of it but when mentioning this to a friend she, very lovingly, confided in me that she was concerned that my son was showing other signs of autism. From there we went to the pediatrician who brushed it off as it being "normal" for kids (boys especially) to not be talking at 18 months and "normal" for little ones to run on their toes, not like to get their hands/feet dirty, not eat, have separation anxiety, chew on everything and to like to bounce, rock and even bang their heads on things…

Even though I wanted so badly to accept this explanation and move on I knew in my heart something wasn't right so I begged for a referral to BabyNet which is a state run program in South Carolina that provides an EI (Early Interventionist), PT, OT, ABA therapy and any other services the child needs for free until the age of 3, for children who qualify. A case worker came to our home and evaluated him in five different areas (he scored low in 3 of the 5) and from there we were assigned an EI. The EI comes to our house once a week and works with my son. She also makes all of the referrals for additional therapies. My son now receives OT twice per week and is in a feeding group with other little guys like him where they work on negotiating textures. He is also going to be starting speech later this month. His verbal communication has increased dramatically since last fall but he still tends to parrot a lot vs. initiating conversation e.g. I'll ask him a question and he will repeat the question back to me…not always, but a lot.

The OTs we work with at the CDS (Center for Developmental Services) were the ones to formally diagnose him with SPD and severe oral defensiveness (he's 2½ and still can't eat from a fork or spoon).

We have an appointment with Developmental Peds later this month to determine if he needs to see a neurologist and have an MRI because he has intention tremors. Also at that appointment they will do a prelim evaluation to determine where he needs to be on the waiting list for his big screening where they will determine if he will be diagnosed with Autism, ADHD, ADD etc.

2. How has this impacted your child's/family's lives?

It has impacted our lives a lot. We are in therapy four times a week and when we are at home we try to take every opportunity we can to work with him.

3. Do you feel you have a good support system? What could improve a parent's support system?

I feel like we have a wonderful support system. My husband and I work well together and his OTs and EI have become people who I consider friends. Even our five year old daughter knows that every time she plays with her brother is an opportunity to help him learn and grow.

I am also LOVING the online support group I have found on Facebook. Reading others' struggles, successes and advice has really helped.

4. What has been the best advice and/or treatment you have heard or tried so far?

One of the methods his OT uses in his eating therapy is to ask him to kiss his food or to blow on it. Getting the food up to the mouth is half the battle…   He has since added cheese and raisins to his limited diet (normally salty/crunchy palate). I have also found weighted blankets, vest, lap pads etc. to be a huge help in calming him down.

5. What has been the most difficult part of your child's diagnosis and what would make it easier for you?

The hardest part has been accepting it. One minute your think you have a normal, healthy 18 month old and then all of a sudden all of these symptoms and behaviors come out of nowhere. Some people swear that it's vaccine related (specifically the MMR vaccine) but I will say that I feel confident that is not true because I waited, out of fear with both of my children, to get them MMR until they were between 20-24 months and saw no change afterwards. My son's behaviors and symptoms were already present by then.

6. How has your child's diagnosis affected them/yourself socially and emotionally?

My little guy is only 2½ years old so he doesn't know any better. As for me, since "coming out" with his diagnosis I have noticed that people are a little bit afraid of him. This year when we tried go out to dinner for our anniversary none of my friends or normal sitters could or would watch the kids for us. I was really hurt by that. I must have called 15 people (all of whom I have kept kids for at one point or another). I know people are busy but some of their excuses were really lame. "I have to wash my car"… give me a break.

7. Has your child's school been supportive or helpful and how? Do you have 504 plan or IEP?

My little guy isn't in elementary school yet but his preschool has been great about letting the EI come into the classroom on weeks when she can't see him at our home. She has started the application process to get him into 3K (when he turns 3) which is offered through the school system. He will get to go from 8. 11 M-F and have access to PT, OT and speech therapy every day.

8. Has there been a positive outcome from your child's diagnosis?

I think so. Early intervention is the key and everyone working with him seems to feel that his progress has been tremendous and that by the time he is ready to start 5K he will be able to be in a regular classroom and handle what is expected from him.

9. What would you like the general public to know about this situation?

I don't think a lot of people know about SPD. Autism and ADHD are everywhere so just getting that recognition and general understanding would be good.

10. If there is anything else you would like to share with our readers on the

subject, not included above, please add it here.

Rachel

Prescott Valley, AZ, USA

1. When did you first notice your child had Sensory Processing Disorder?

When and how was he/she officially diagnosed?

We noticed sensory issues at 6 months but she was not officially diagnosed until she was 3 years old. The therapist was hoping she would grow out of it but it looks like she will have sensory for a while.

2. How has this impacted your child's/family's lives?

It has impacted the family in many ways but we are a close knit family and work together to make everything work well. My child knows she has issues different to other children and is okay with it and actually very proud to be the person she is!

3. Do you feel you have a good support system? What could improve a

parent's support system?

I have a strong support system, our extended family is also close knit. My sister helped me pay for my daughter's SPIOs, my sister in law made her weighted blankets, and cousins and my mom help me find more information on SPD.

4. What has been the best advice and/or treatment you have heard or tried

so far?

The SPIOs was the best thing the therapist could have told me about! That and finding ways to meet her needs at home when she is having a bad day (spinning in the computer chair while wrapped in a weighted blanket)!

5. What has been the most difficult part of your child's diagnosis and what

would make it easier for you?

The most difficult part of the diagnosis is her realizing she cannot sit still as long as other children and telling her teachers so. She has been working on attention but it would be easier if teachers would help me with ideas instead of just telling me she is disrupting the class with her yelling and running around during sitting time.

6. How has your child's diagnosis affected them/yourself socially and emotionally?

It hasn't affected us for the most part unless she is having a bad day. I get emotionally drained trying to help her on those bad days. For the most part I like to find ways we can have fun no matter what anyone else around us thinks. My children are most important to me and deserve my full attention and support!

7. Has your child's school been supportive or helpful and how? Do you have 504 plan or IEP?

My daughter has an IEP - last year I was called daily with issues in class. This year she has been moved to a sensory room so we are very hopeful of working more closely with the teacher and getting some good ideas!

8. Has there been a positive outcome from your child's diagnosis?

A positive outcome from her diagnosis is that I have ways to help her now, rather than just throw up my hands and not know what to do. She is a positive child and always happy and her diagnosis helped me understand what she is going through and what makes her who she is!

9. What would you like the general public to know about this situation?

I can only do my part in spreading SPD awareness but I would like the public to not be so judgmental about parents in public. I have actually helped other parents with children acting out in public because it is embarrassing to have people tell me how bad a parent I am when it has nothing to do with my parenting.

Cassandra I. Coleman

Gresham, Oregon

1. When did you first notice your child had Sensory Processing Disorder? When and how was he/she officially diagnosed?

At two days old I noticed there was something going on with my son, and by age two weeks I knew for sure. I did my research and by the time he was a month old I knew it had to be SPD and/or Autism. My husband and I took him to many doctors and specialists and by age four months he was diagnosed with SPD by the Early Childhood program where we lived at the time. They did an in-home evaluation of him and began weekly services shortly afterwards.

2. How has this impacted your child's/family's lives?

I could write a book on how SPD has impacted our lives, including my son's. In fact I have blogged, to some degree, from my pregnancy all the way to the present day about my son and what we've been through. My son just turned 3 last month, July 15, and the first year and a half were the hardest on me and us as a family. Luckily my husband and I have a solid relationship and while it's been hard with our son, I feel it's only made us stronger as a couple. Our daughter is 11, and it's been hard on her as well, but she's a great big sister and she's done an amazing job with her brother.

3. Do you feel you have a good support system? What could improve a parent's support system?

Yes! I do, but I think I need more. I don't have any friends around me, and that makes it hard. I haven't been able to get out and join any groups and I feel that's an important factor for us as parents to be able to make it through the challenges we face. I have a lot of online support, but the actual presence of people and their support is very different.

4. What has been the best advice and/or treatment you have heard or tried
so far?

It's really hard to say because what works one day, may not work the next, or even in the same day. I think the greatest thing about meeting people and being able to have open communication with them online is being able to talk about stuff like this. I love the fact that we can post our concerns or ask for help or ideas, and there are so many different people who have been through it, or who are also looking for the same kinds of answers. As for what has helped, several different things at different times, but I feel that brushing alone has been a huge help for my son.

5. What has been the most difficult part of your child's diagnosis and what
would make it easier for you?

Well, in the beginning, his first year and a half, it was really hard on me and I did everything I could to learn what I needed to in order to make sure my son was taken care of in the best way possible. Now that I've accept him for who he is and what he deals with, it's been easier on me, but that doesn't mean life is "easy". I think what is the most difficult for me is the fact that I am with him all day and night, and I don't get that many breaks away from my son. So, more breaks to breathe and refresh before having to be around my son again would be VERY helpful to me.

6. How has your child's diagnosis affected them/yourself socially
and emotionally?

Well, sadly, since having my son I have developed anxiety and agoraphobia, and that is a whole new world for me! I've always been a social butterfly, so to now be afraid of social situations just breaks my heart. This person that I am, was not the person that I was before having my son. I am working all the time with my therapist and husband to get through this, but I would have to say that is the biggest impact on my life. Since I am not able to get out and be around people, it also means that my son doesn't either. I feel terrible about this, but my therapist assures me that my son is doing great. At first I was devastated over this baby that I had in my arms that just screamed all the time, instead of the baby I thought I was going to have. It took me a lot of time to come to terms with what we were dealing with, and I did my research to learn about everything I possibly could in order to help my son, and to help myself feel better that at least I was able to help him even if the doctors we had seen couldn't. Thankfully now we are in a great area and the care team that he has is doing a great job with him.

7. *Has your child's school been supportive or helpful and how? Do you have 504 plan or IEP?*

My son isn't in school yet, and it's a subject that we talk about a lot, and are working on with his behavior therapist. I'm terrified to send him to school, because I was a teacher in many different places and I know what goes on "behind the scenes" and what kind of lies are told to parents, and I refuse to allow that to happen to my son. So I'm really torn now that I have a special needs son who will at some point in his life have to go to school. I am trying to work myself up to this point and hopefully we can get him into some kind of part time program that will help both of us transition into a school setting. In the meantime time I am my son's teacher and I'm perfectly happy with that.

8. *Has there been a positive outcome from your child's diagnosis?*

A positive outcome from his diagnosis? Hmmm…… I'm not really sure how to answer this one. I think for me, since I am so well in tune with my children, I was able to see something wasn't right when my son was just two days old so I don't really feel like his diagnosis has had any kind of outcome for our family. I feel like the only positive outcome that happened was when doctors started listening to me and seeing what I was telling them was going on. Other than that I'm really not sure what else I could say has been a positive outcome. Maybe what has changed in me? My daughter has always been an easy, calm, and very much "normal" child, she and my son are complete opposites, sharing only their affectionate manner in common. The change in me, or what I've realized, is my ability to handle my son, and he's taught me so much by just being him. At some point I was able to switch from being sad over what he was going through, to being able to tune into him to see what makes him work, and what I can do to work WITH him. So I guess the positive outcome is the way I was able to switch how I viewed my son, and now see him in a different way than I did a year and a half ago.

9. *What would you like the general public to know about this situation?*

There is a LOT that they should know. Sadly though, people won't learn if they don't have an interest. Most people who don't have special needs kids won't even care to hear about what we all go through. There are some people who will take the time to learn some of this stuff, but only because they are connected to someone who has SPD. I feel that there isn't really one particular aspect that is more important than another, but maybe as a whole the general public need to learn compassion and understanding. There are so many judgmental people out there, and it's the looks and the whispered comments, or even the unasked for "advice" from people that make parents of special needs kids nervous or upset. Often times the best thing to do is not stare but offer a comment of understanding. When I've gone out in public with or without my son, I often think that the people around make it harder on me and my husband by staring, or making comments. Instead I would feel so much better if there were comments such as "I understand what you're going through", "I've had to deal with the same thing", or "You're doing a great job with your child". Something kind and encouraging always makes things easier on a person.

10. *If there is anything else you would like to share with our readers on the subject, not included above, please add it here.*

1. When did you first notice your child had Sensory Processing Disorder? When and how was he/she officially diagnosed?

She was 15 months old when I first noticed sensory issues (I am a chiropractor) but prior to that we stopped hitting milestones and she never liked tummy time, didn't creep or crawl and didn't walk until PT and only then at 22 - 23 months. We put her in a special needs daycare - that helped. SPD isn't a formal diagnosis yet in Tennesee and we have been to Vandy Children's Developmental many times!

2. How has this impacted your child's/family's lives?

We are significantly behind in development. We have very little support and are extremely tired. No one wants to babysit, so lots of things that would strengthen or help with our marriage get ignored. We have had to seek out support groups. We have tried activities such as dance with a mommy and me class which she loved but has already, at the age of 4, discovered how cruel adults can be. We are very very scheduled with EVERYTHING!!

3. Do you feel you have a good support system? What could improve a parent's support system?

No, we have no support other than a special needs ministry group we have found. We have no family support.

4. What has been the best advice and/or treatment you have heard or tried so far?

Weighted blanket. Our school system has great special needs programing and we have wonderful therapies. Best advice - ADVOCATE for your child and their needs

5. What has been the most difficult part of your child's diagnosis and what would make it easier for you?

That we lost a lot of family/friends due to them denying or not understanding or just plain shutting us out. You can't make that easier, but the thing I would love is more special needs activities!!

6. How has your child's diagnosis affected them/yourself socially and emotionally?

Us more than her, she doesn't know she is different really because we have managed to catch it and cater to her needs and teach her how to cater for herself as well. Socially, we are at home with a 4 year old all the time, so of course we feel like no one understands our situation!! See above answers.

7. Has your child's school been supportive or helpful and how? Do you have 504 plan or IEP?

We are in a special needs PreK we have a great school system and have lots of therapies there. We also have an IEP.

8. Has there been a positive outcome from your child's diagnosis?

We are making progress…

9. What would you like the general public to know about this situation?

That it isn't the parent's fault, it isn't anyone's fault, the child isn't spoiled, the child isn't misbehaving and no the child isn't a brat just because they don't want to socialize or touch you. Sometimes they just need to know you better.

10. *If there is anything else you would like to share with our readers on the subject, not included above, please add it here.*

Please, please, please educate yourselves and think before speaking. These kiddos understand more than you think or give them credit for and are easily hurt. Their family members are also hurt by your lack of education.

Julie Foser

Buffalo, NY, United States

1. When did you first notice your child had Sensory Processing Disorder? When and how was he/she officially diagnosed?

I noticed something was wrong with my son, Jayden right from birth. He appeared to be healthy and you would not notice anything was wrong from seeing him in person. He does not have a visible disability. But from birth, he cried day and night almost as if he was in pain. I knew as a mother that something was wrong, but everyone just thought I was over reacting. People had suggestions, but I already tried everything they mentioned. I felt helpless, not being able to comfort my baby. I took him to the doctor many times. They tested him for allergies, switched his formula, he was put on medicine for acid reflux. My son continued to cry all day and all night. It was difficult on his father and me. We switched shifts staying up with him, without ever getting a good night's rest. You could hear him screaming in the background, so unless you were to the point of exhaustion you could not sleep anyway. As a parent it is a natural reaction to want to hold and comfort your baby. He did not want to be picked up - when we picked him up, he cried more. Nothing seemed to work. I felt completely helpless, and just kept trying to find ways to comfort him. I learned that he did not like being held, he wanted to be swaddled tightly and left alone.

When he was about one year old, he started head banging, hitting, punching, biting, scratching, pounding and throwing things, throwing himself on the floor, and had serious meltdowns and tantrums consistently throughout each day. He never wanted to go near people; in fact he would run away. He would scream if you held his hand, or tried to pick him up. He hated straps on highchairs and strollers. He screamed at the top of his lungs, even worse in public places and stores. The head banging was my biggest concern; I kept taking him to the doctors, they said he would outgrow it. Well, one day he touched my stove and he did not jump. The stove was hot; when I touched it I jumped. This is the day

I realized there was something seriously wrong. I contacted agencies, and they evaluated him.

When I saw the evaluation, I was shocked. I knew right away that they knew what they were doing. In fact, during the deep pressure massage and song, his body relaxed. He literally sighed and had a look of relief in his little blue eyes. I had tears in my eyes. I knew without words that they knew what was wrong. He was diagnosed first with Sensory Processing Disorder and was then was put on a waiting list for an Autism evaluation, which took about a year to get. He was finally tested at 3 years old and diagnosed with PDD-NOS, which is on the Autism spectrum. He has had approximately 15 - 20 total evaluations from different specialists, doctors and psychologists throughout the past three years.

2. How has this impacted your child's/family's lives?

There are many difficult moments, and challenging days. Our lives have not been the same since the day he was born. My family life at home has definitely changed. We stay home a lot more. We have teachers and specialists in our house 3 hours per day, 5 days a week. Although it is very stressful at times, I can't say that everything changed for the worse. Each little milestone for him is a huge deal for us. We all worked hard with him to get him to the point he is at now. My little Jayden has the most amazing sense of humor. He can make us laugh so hard; we love watching him dance and sing. He loves cars, trains, planes, coloring, bingo dotters, books, music and painting.

3. Do you feel you have a good support system? What could improve a parent's support system?

We have.

4. What has been the best advice and/or treatment you have heard or tried so far?

The two best treatments are the deep pressure massage and the weighted backpack he carries. We tell him what we will be doing next before doing whatever it is. This helps him with transition. In public places, I bring him headphones and music to help drown out the noises that overwhelm him. Since he likes smashing things, I bought him a tool table to pound on. I purchased a beanbag chair for him to jump on, punch, and cuddle into. The beanbag chair has been very helpful.

5. What has been the most difficult part of your child's diagnosis and what would make it easier for you?

The most difficult part of my son's diagnosis is the head banging and the behavioral issues. I am not sure what would make this easier for me, other than hoping that through our patience, love and prayer that he will be able to cope better with this disorder.

6. How has your child's diagnosis affected them/yourself socially and emotionally?

Jayden's diagnosis has affected our social lives in many ways. We don't get many visitors. Some people have actually asked us not to come around unless we get a babysitter. Obviously, with his diagnosis, finding a sitter is not easy, and not cheap either! Throughout the three years I have experienced so many emotions. The day he was diagnosed, I was happy that we finally had answers and could figure out a plan to try to help him. I was also sad to find out that there was something wrong with my baby, and I couldn't do anything to make it go away. There was no medicine, cast or magical Band-Aid to make it better. There are many difficult days and many days I feel alone in the fight for my son. Every day that goes by, I have to remind myself to stay strong, and hold it together for my entire family. I am the strong one, or so they think. Each and every day, I hold all of my tears inside and just keep moving forward.

7. Has your child's school been supportive or helpful and how? Do you have 504 plan or IEP?

My son has an IEP for now. His teachers have been amazing. They have put up with a lot and helped not only him, but me too. I raised my older son, but never a child with a disability. I was clueless and without them, I might still be. He will soon be going to a school for Autistic children and they will be working on ABA with him at school. We will be continuing services for 3 hours a day at home, with new teachers. We will be sad to see his Early Intervention teachers go. They are here so much, they seem like they are part of our family. We are looking forward to his new pre-K services and hope that we can work together to help my little man.

8. Has there been a positive outcome from your child's diagnosis?

My son has made many improvements over the past year with help from his teachers. I work with him each day and they have told me that they can tell that I spend a lot of time with him. He is considered high functioning and there is hope that through services that he may be able to function in a regular school. We will not know until that time. This is not a promise, and I am aware of that, but I just stay positive and hopeful.

9. What would you like the general public to know about this situation?

The biggest thing I would like to tell the general public is that you cannot visibly see Sensory Processing Disorder or PDD-NOS. When you see a child throwing a fit, try not to judge or make faces and rude comments. Just because a child is acting up does not mean the parents are "bad parents". In fact, the parents that I have met that have children with these diagnoses have more patience and love than you can ever imagine. The other thing I would like to tell the general public is that sensory processing is common in children on the Autism spectrum. Just because a child does not look like the severely affected autistic kids, does not mean that they don't have it. That is why they call it the "Autism Spectrum".

I should not have to explain to rude people that my son is disabled. I don't want him to hear that every day. I am trying my hardest to help a high functioning Autistic child with sensory processing disorder. We have heard there is hope for us. I am not asking for help, just keep those thoughts in mind when you see the parents struggling with their kids. You never know if the child has a medical condition and what the parents do to help them each and every day. You may not have the patience to hear it for a few minutes, but we work with them, love them and care for them every single day of our lives.

10. *If there is anything else you would like to share with our readers on the subject, not included above, please add it here.*

I just wanted to add that I do have a 14 year old, named Brandon. He is smart, healthy, plays sports and is an amazing brother and son. He is very understanding, helpful, loving and caring towards his little brother. My life would not be complete without the two of them.

Jo Miller

Denver, Colorado USA

1. When did you first notice your child had Sensory Processing Disorder?

When and how was he/she officially diagnosed?

I noticed my son had something going on since birth. Didn't know what it was until I found out about SPD a year ago, he was diagnosed recently at age 6.

2. How has this impacted your child's/family's lives?

It has been a great struggle in our home because it limits a lot of what we can do, where we can go or who watches him. Family doesn't understand which causes us a lot of grief. It has also been a great struggle making decisions about where to get his education.

3. Do you feel you have a good support system? What could improve a

parent's support system?

Our support system could be better if teachers where more educated about SPD and how to handle it. I think the schools need more individual support for these kids. Also I think if families would accept and learn more about it instead of resisting the diagnosis. Also, I have struggled to find a local support group for the families, where kids could meet other kids with SPD and parents could support each other.

4. What has been the best advice and/or treatment you have heard or tried

so far?

We are in the beginning phases, don't know what might work yet, but the best thing I heard was from a friend, the OT who did the initial evaluation. She said they call kids like mine "bump and crash" kids. I was so happy to hear this was normal for kids with SPD. I felt validated that I wasn't just another "bad parent".

5. What has been the most difficult part of your child's diagnosis and what would make it easier for you?

The diagnosis is great, gives us a starting point for treatment, but when you try to explain to someone what it is, they have never heard of it. It's not like autism where they immediately "get it" because they hear so much about it. We need awareness!

6. How has your child's diagnosis affected them/yourself socially and emotionally?

Socially/emotionally I feel isolated. He doesn't act like his peers or my friends' kids. We feel different and judged by people don't understand.

7. Has your child's school been supportive or helpful and how? Do you have 504 plan or IEP?

We have neither at the moment but may have IEP for upcoming school year. His teachers try to understand but lack the time and energy needed to give individually needed support.

8. Has there been a positive outcome from your child's diagnosis?

The only positive outcome so far (diagnosis was only 4 months ago) is validation and a new attitude of patience from me.

9. What would you like the general public to know about this situation?

I would love to have more awareness - the more people know the more they will react with patience and compassion instead of judgmental ignorant attitudes.

10. If there is anything else you would like to share with our readers on the subject, not included above, please add it here.

I was told that in the US, doctors could not officially diagnose SPD or say anything about it in paperwork because it would jeopardize the insurance and nothing would be covered. That is sad. If more research was done and a general acknowledgement from the medical community, there would be more help for these kids.

Jennifer S.

West Bloomfield, MI USA

1. *When did you first notice your child had Sensory Processing Disorder? When and how was he/she officially diagnosed?*

I've known that my daughter, who is now 10 years old, has had "sensory issues" since she was very little. She was finally diagnosed when she was 9½ years old by an occupational therapist. It was recommended by a therapist she was seeing at the time, who asked last October (2012) if she had ever had an evaluation for autism or sensory processing disorder. I went home and looked up information on Sensory Processing Disorder. It was unreal how much it sounded like what my daughter has. I called my friend who has a daughter with the same thing to find out what diagnosis code to use so the services and evaluation would be covered by insurance. She gave me the information and I called the pediatrician the next day to have her write a prescription for me with the codes and diagnosis given to me by my friend.

2. *How has this impacted your child's/family's lives?*

It has made me more understanding of some of my daughter's and son's behaviors and why they do things that they do. For instance my son, who was just diagnosed last May (2013), won't wear anything except sweat pants or sweat shorts. I can now see and understand why my daughter might have a meltdown when we are at a place she wanted to go in the first place like Chuck E. Cheese or Zap Zone.

3. *Do you feel you have a good support system? What could improve a parent's support system?*

Nope! My in-laws tell me all the time there is nothing wrong with my daughter - that she behaves the way she does because I don't discipline her. My daughter is now on anti-depressant meds because of the way my father-in-law treats and talks to her. It was a nightmare when I was working full-time and he was having to take care of my kids. My father-in-law told my daughter's OT that she didn't need to go for therapy. He had to take her one week when her Dad and I were both working. He is so frustrating to deal with that I have no choice to ignore him since it is an unending battle. I do happen to have a couple of friends that have kids with the same diagnosis or special needs. I can either email or Facebook them if I have any questions or need to vent. The "Sensory Processing Disorder Parent Support Group" page on Facebook has been a huge support system for me. I can read about other kiddos on the page that are the same as my two kids and it makes me feel better knowing I am not the only one on the planet with kids like this.

4. What has been the best advice and/or treatment you have heard or tried so far?

Weekly occupational therapy and purchasing a weighted blanket for my daughter. I wish we could get one for my son too, but I was laid off from my job since we got my daughter's blanket.

5. What has been the most difficult part of your child's diagnosis and what would make it easier for you?

The most difficult part is trying to get my daughter tested for other things such as Auditory Processing Disorder, Neuropsych testing, and testing for autism. The insurance company will not cover any of the testing since my daughter is 10 years old and they stopped covering APD testing within the last year. I tried getting her tested two years ago for this and I was told she had mild conductive hearing loss in both ears and so they couldn't complete it. Now it's not covered at all. It's so incredibly frustrating!!

6. How has your child's diagnosis affected them/yourself socially and emotionally?

The diagnosis itself hasn't really changed anything. My daughter still has socialization issues like she did before. It has just better explained the way my daughter and son operate. I now understand why they are the way they are. I have not been that open with family and friends unless it is someone that totally understands what this disorder is about. I get negative reactions from some people, so for me it's not worth trying to explain. The few people I have told, like my own Mom, still get upset at my daughter when she bumps into her or starts eating with her hands. I have explained to Mom that it is one of the issues to do with the SPD and dyspraxia but she doesn't get it. She tells me that it should be taught in our home. OMG! It has been numerous times!

7. Has your child's school been supportive or helpful and how? Do you have

504 plan or IEP?

The school has been very supportive! My daughter now has an IEP, but they don't recognize SPD in any public school system in the state of Michigan, so her IEP is very basic in what it states should be implemented at school such as no timed tests and allowing my daughter extra time on assignments and a modified homework program to reduce frustration. She was already using the resource room long before the IEP was written, but that was also one of the recommendations. I have given her teachers at school some articles about SPD and Dyspraxia to read. A couple of them either called and emailed me back stating they couldn't believe how much my daughter sounds like the child/children in the articles. I was able to request that my son NOT have a specific teacher this coming school year based on his diagnosis of SPD. I brought a letter written by my daughter's OT that suggests certain personality traits of teachers that my two children should or should not have.

8. Has there been a positive outcome from your child's diagnosis?

The positive thing about the diagnosis is helping us (her parents) understand her better and it also has helped her teachers at school be more understanding with some of her quirks.

9. What would you like the general public to know about this situation?

I wish that Sensory Processing Disorder was more well-known like ADHD and Autism diagnoses are. Most people have never heard of Sensory Processing Disorder and some that have don't believe it is a disorder. If they put out flyers on the disorder in pediatricians offices that might help people understand better. I can always find flyers on ADHD and similar diagnoses.

10. If there is anything else you would like to share with our readers on the subject, not included above, please add it here.

Angie Carlozzi

Ocala, USA

1. When did you first notice your child had Sensory Processing Disorder? When and how was he/she officially diagnosed?

He was always very quiet and hardly cried as an infant. Since he was my first, I thought he was just a really good baby. As he got older I started to notice things that concerned me. If he was playing or watching TV, he was oblivious to me calling his name. I thought he might having a hearing impairment. He never cried when getting vaccines and he would sometimes tantrum for no reason at all, or so I thought. One day he hit his head pretty hard and had a huge bump but he didn't cry. That was when I knew something was wrong. He was officially diagnosed at 2½ years old. He received a developmental evaluation by an early start program and then was evaluated by a pediatric occupational therapist.

2. How has this impacted your child's/family's lives?

Getting a diagnosis was met with mixed emotions. I was so relieved to finally have answers, but at the same time my heart was breaking over the idea that something was officially "wrong" with my child. I racked my brain trying to figure out if I did something wrong during the pregnancy. Did I eat healthy enough? Did I avoid enough stress? You eventually realize that it's not your fault, but that comes much later.

3. Do you feel you have a good support system? What could improve a parent's support system?

When he was first diagnosed my family felt that it was just a label and that he would outgrow it. Some thought it was an excuse for his "bad" behavior. With patience, determination and constantly having to educate others, my family now understands and is supportive. They accommodate our needs as best they can.

4. What has been the best advice and/or treatment you have heard or tried

so far?

Don't try to fix your child. Embrace your child's uniqueness, remind yourself of all their positive qualities and praise them for it. Approach treatment with the intent of helping your child to be comfortable with themselves. He or she may never be like every other child and that is ok. A combination of Occupational Therapy and Massage Therapy worked wonders for us. The main thing is we give him the tools he needs to be comfortable - headphones, chewies, fidgets and stress reducing techniques.

5. What has been the most difficult part of your child's diagnosis and what

would make it easier for you?

Knowing when to push him further or to take a step back and be ok with where he is at. It's a constant juggle between encouragement and enabling. I'm not sure what would make this easier. You want to push as hard as you can so that he can be independent and safe in all environments, but you don't want to push too hard.

6. How has your child's diagnosis affected them/yourself socially

and emotionally?

He has always had a difficult time making friends but the ones that he has are great. He understands that he is different but not disabled, just differently abled. As for us parents, we adopted more understanding friends. Ones that don't mind him tuning out with his headphones and don't judge during a meltdown. Ones that understand that having a child limits the amount of time that we can talk or hang out, having one with SPD limits it even more. The same applied to families. The ones that didn't want to be supportive were cut out of our lives. Emotionally it has ups and downs. You worry a little more, ok, a lot more. At the same time you have an amazing bond with your child that I think parents of neurotypical children might miss out on.

7. Has your child's school been supportive or helpful and how? Do you have

504 plan or IEP?

We had an IEP until second grade. The school was somewhat supportive. Since he had a lot of early intervention, his SPD did not affect him too greatly in school. He only needed a few accommodations. It really depended on his teachers. We had some great ones that wanted to learn and help him grow and a couple that thought the label was an excuse.

8. Has there been a positive outcome from your child's diagnosis?

Thanks to his early diagnosis we were able to get him lots of help and he is doing really great. Mainly, it empowered us to be able to help our child and make us realize we weren't bad parents.

9. What would you like the general public to know about this situation?

Try to put yourself in their shoes before passing judgment. Everyone has some form of sensory issues. You may not like the sound of a metal fork scraping across the plate or the sound of nails on a chalkboard. For someone with sensory processing disorder this could be anything - the flushing of the toilet, the humming of the refrigerator, the sound of someone tapping a pencil can all be too much. For them it's like someone blasting the sound of nails on a chalkboard from a huge stereo directly against your ear only they don't shut it off. Would you be able to concentrate or be polite in that situation? Probably not and that is only considering the auditory side of it.

10. If there is anything else you would like to share with our readers on the

subject, not included above, please add it here.

I would love to see more programs for siblings with children affected by SPD. Siblings have to take a back seat sometimes for their diagnosed siblings needs. It can be very stressful for them.

To parents who do not have a child with special needs, PLEASE do not try to act like an expert based on a few articles you read on Google. Offer an ear, ask all the questions you want, but don't try to fix it ;) Our kids are

very cool; they are just extra sensitive and maybe a little clumsy. Their
brains are just wired differently.

1. *When did you first notice your child had Sensory Processing Disorder? When and how was he/she officially diagnosed?*

Our son came to us through the foster care system. I have been an exceptional education teacher for 18 years and I noticed symptoms immediately upon him arriving in our home. He was officially diagnosed at a little over three years old.

2. *How has this impacted your child's/family's lives?*

His diagnosis impacts our lives daily! We have to constantly fight our instinctual responses of wanting to set consequences. He needs constant reminders, re-teaching, positive examples and statements, and freedom to be himself (even sitting on the couch on his head). He needs to know it is ok to be himself. At the same time, we have to teach his little brother that it is ok for his brother to think differently than he does.

3. *Do you feel you have a good support system? What could improve a parent's support system?*

I don't feel we have a very good support system. The diagnosis itself isn't even readily acknowledged in the medical field and the educational system. He is often considered to be ADHD due to the hyperactive behavior that he exhibits from seeking sensory stimulation. We as parents need to do a better job of educating those around us and our son. We need to do a better job supporting one another. Finding a babysitter is nearly impossible. They rarely come back after an evening with him.

4. What has been the best advice and/or treatment you have heard or tried

so far?

Best treatment: occupational therapy that addresses his specific sensory needs. We also use essential oils, compression shirts, and weighted blankets/vests/lap pad.

Best advice: educate yourself, be patient and understanding.

5. What has been the most difficult part of your child's diagnosis and what

would make it easier for you?

Most difficult part is education. It is very challenging to get educational staff to understand he isn't a "bad" kid and much of what he does is for sensory input (running into people, crashing into things). Our son happens to also have a lot of learning difficulties so it makes it even more challenging.

6. How has your child's diagnosis affected them/yourself socially

and emotionally?

It has had a big impact on all of us socially. We are rarely invited over to other homes for play dates. He tends to break a lot of toys and can inadvertently hurt others with his sensory seeking. He doesn't truly play with other children. Most of his play is parallel play but not true interaction. Kids will often "give up" on interacting with him when he doesn't respond. He will often just keep running and running and the kids get tired of trying to get him to stop to talk to them.

7. Has your child's school been supportive or helpful and how? Do you have

504 plan or IEP?

We have an IEP for our son. As an exceptional education teacher I knew what to fight for. We have yet to find staff to accept and understand the sensory delays and not just blame it on bad behavior. We are hoping for a better year this year since we are moving him to the school I work at.

8. Has there been a positive outcome from your child's diagnosis?

Positive outcomes:

- learning to be thankful daily for what we have
- increased education
- unique qualities in him that will one day be seen as assets instead of a disability

9. What would you like the general public to know about this situation?

I would like the public to know that when you see a child throwing a fit, being really loud or falling down in public it doesn't mean the parents are "too lenient" or the child is "out of control". I would like the public to know that my son has talents. I would like them to know that he wants to have friends. I would like them to know that we are lonely and need friends. I would like them to know that our son is VERY special and has a lot to offer the world if people would just take the time to learn how he ticks!

10. If there is anything else you would like to share with our readers on the subject, not included above, please add it here.

I feel like this is almost a silent disorder. Other than atypical behavior, our kids look "normal." Please don't pass judgments on parents when you see them struggling with a child's behavior.

Rebecca Waldron

Wolverhampton, West Midlands, England

1. When did you first notice your child had Sensory Processing Disorder? When and how he/she was officially diagnosed?

Since birth Millie always had issues with sleep, kisses, cuddles, certain clothes etc. but it came to a head at the age of around 4½ years.

I had spoken to the doctor previously and no diagnosis was forthcoming. I did some research myself and discovered information on tactile defensiveness. I told the doctor that I thought this was what she had, he referred her to OT who confirmed Millie does have Sensory Modulation Disorder.

2. How has this impacted your child's/family's lives?

For the first five years of her life Millie did not sleep through the night even once. She would wake regularly, often up to ten times a night. She would cry during the night with pains in her legs and as a baby she would flex and stretch her legs while crying. This had an obvious impact on her father and I, our health and relationship suffered.

At times of change/transition e.g. end of the school year, holidays, and new school term etc., Millie develops serious issues with her socks, pants, seams and labels in clothes. She has gone weeks during the summer without wearing shoes, preferring to go barefoot or wear slippers. She becomes distraught when she needs to wear clothes and I can tell it does physically hurt her. She does not understand why she feels like this when no-one else does and she will become upset or frustrated with herself.

This affects the family as we are limited in activities and days out/holidays we can enjoy. Millie's younger sister misses out on activities during the holidays and she has, on occasion, copied her sister and refused to wear socks etc.

3. Do you feel you have a good support system? What could improve a

parent's support system?

I feel as though the disorder is not taken very seriously by family members and doctors alike. The OT was very supportive with regular phone calls as we waited months for an appointment. I think SPD should be brought into the public consciousness as quite often I have heard or read that it is believed to be a product of poor upbringing rather than an actual psychological condition.

4. What has been the best advice and/or treatment you have heard or tried

so far?

I won a weighted blanket for my daughter and it has changed our lives. She has slept through every night since we received it around four months ago. This coupled with a deep pressure brushing technique shown by the OT has been amazing. Many people have commented on the change in Millie and on her increased confidence.

5. What has been the most difficult part of your child's diagnosis and what

would make it easier for you?

Actually finding out what the disorder was. The doctor had no idea and I felt as though I was not taken entirely seriously. I felt like an over-anxious parent.

6. How has your child's diagnosis affected them/yourself socially

and emotionally?

Socially Millie has always appeared standoffish with family members/friends when refusing to hug/kiss them. This has often resulted in uncomfortable discussions and opinions from others who do not understand how she feels. Certain activities in the playground will be avoided as physical contact makes her uncomfortable, this can put strain on her friendships. When Millie is going through a difficult phase, she appears constantly tense and tightly wound, this can manifest itself in meltdowns, unreasonable anger and frustration.

We have had to refuse certain social events due to Millie's inability to wear clothes at one time or another.

There are always those, family and friends, who do not put much stock in psychological disorders and are skeptical, this can lead to tension.

I have suffered myself with anxiety and depression for a number of years, the lack of sleep for so long and the worry and stress at times has not helped with these conditions. My relationship with my partner has been irretrievably damaged due to my state of mental health.

7. Has your child's school been supportive or helpful and how? Do you have 504 plan or IEP?

Millie's class teacher has assured us she will do all she can do help Millie feel comfortable at school and was very keen to find out about the disorder. The school itself has not followed up on her diagnosis and has not implemented any changes or developed a statement for her as far as I am aware.

8. Has there been a positive outcome from your child's diagnosis?

Yes, in the fact that I know I am not being over-anxious, that I can put a name to what is wrong and that I know there are others out there who are experiencing the same issue. The weighted blanket and brushing technique have really been an absolute godsend.

Even though I have a diagnosis, I still have to argue for its existence with family members, friends and even my partner, who remains skeptical. Many still believe Millie is just a "difficult child".

9. What would you like the general public to know about this situation?

I would like there to be more information for the general public regarding SPD. It is hard for people to understand if they have not experienced it first hand and with their own child. I KNEW something wasn't right with Millie, I KNEW it was hurting her to wear socks/pants, I KNEW she was so frustrated with herself that it couldn't have been "put on", yet I couldn't say for sure that if it wasn't my child but another I was observing from the outside, I wouldn't be as disbelieving as others have been in the past with Millie. It is very difficult to promote awareness with such a disorder.

10. If there is anything else you would like to share with our readers on the subject, not included above, please add it here.

Karen Ogden

Quepos Costa Rica

1. When did you first notice your child had Sensory Processing Disorder?

When and how was he/she officially diagnosed?

He was about 2years old. I had him in speech therapy and his therapist told me about SPD.

2. How has this impacted your child's/family's lives?

It has been difficult but now is much easier. I didn't have much support at the beginning so felt very alone. His big sister has had every toy she owned broken by him and has had to make many sacrifices. I have spent three years driving six hours once a week to take him to therapy and that has been financially draining. He's now 5½ years old and is doing much better.

3. Do you feel you have a good support system? What could improve a

parent's support system?

I have an amazing set of therapists that have helped me a lot. When I could no longer financially afford to pay, they dropped their price 75% so I could afford to continue, which was a lifesaver. My husband has come a long way and is now supportive but it took a long time.

4. What has been the best advice and/or treatment you have heard or tried

so far?

Therapeutic Listening – has made an amazing difference in his life. The headphones and music can calm him down. Occupational Therapy is another one that has made the most difference. He has learned about personal spacing, how to regulate himself.

5. What has been the most difficult part of your child's diagnosis and what would make it easier for you?

- Traveling to therapy, we travel 6 hours once a week so he can go.
- Having patience to deal with him on the really bad days when I'm tired.

6. How has your child's diagnosis affected them/yourself socially and emotionally?

When he was young, I didn't like to go places because it was so hard. When he was diagnosed, I posted as much as I could on Facebook about it and friends started to be educated on what he had so they understood better and it became easier.

BEFORE he was diagnosed, we would discipline him for things that he didn't know were wrong. AFTER he was diagnosed, I could see in his eyes when he really didn't have a clue.

7. Has your child's school been supportive or helpful and how? Do you have 504 plan or IEP?

I live in Costa Rica so we do not have plans for school children. His first year in school was hell. His teacher said he was an awful child, a trouble maker and just a bad kid. I fought tooth and nail for the first year. Luckily, he has had two great teachers the past couple years who cared enough to educate themselves on SPD and he is doing well in school.

8. Has there been a positive outcome from your child's diagnosis?

The school is now educated about SPD and able to help other children with SPD instead of just thinking of them as trouble makers.

9. What would you like the general public to know about this situation?

That it is real, it isn't made up or in our minds. These children have real issues.

10. If there is anything else you would like to share with our readers on the subject, not included above, please add it here.

Put articles on Facebook that are easy and short to read for your friends to educate themselves. I think most of them will be "Oh right, now it all makes sense."

You didn't do anything wrong

Therapy, therapy, therapy, it has made such a massive difference in our life, I can't imagine where we would be today without it.

Sydney Platt

Duncan BC, CANADA

1. When did you first notice your child had Sensory Processing Disorder? When and how was he/she officially diagnosed?

She began getting unexplained migraine headaches at the age of 6. In grade 5, she suddenly stated that she wasn't going to go to school anymore because it was too noisy, smelly and made it so she couldn't breathe. She was officially diagnosed at the end of grade 6 when she was aged 11. It was $3500, not covered. We still have no help for her.

2. How has this impacted your child's/family's lives?

Her brother wants nothing to do with her because he thinks I don't discipline her enough. He is mostly at his Dad's now so she really misses her big brother. He gets frustrated with her "messes" and "moods", so doesn't want to be around her. She no longer wants to go to Dad's house, I believe because Dad feels she is "undisciplined" and he has no understanding of her sensitivities. He is a sensory seeker, she is an avoider, so that puts them at opposite ends of the spectrum. It has pulled our family apart and there is no one to help.

3. Do you feel you have a good support system? What could improve a parent's support system?

ABSOLUTELY NOT! There is no support, people don't even acknowledge there is such a thing. Ali was "kicked out" of counselling at the local Ministry of Children because she won't speak (elected mutism). Hello, don't you think that should raise a red flag? So they told me it was pointless for her to go, that she wasn't "ready" for counselling. No one will help her. It's rather disgusting how she is crying out for help and no one will help her.

There is NO support for kids with SPD, unless they are labelled autistic. There is no funding, no extra help at school. Most people, including some professionals, don't even believe there is such a thing.

4. What has been the best advice and/or treatment you have heard or tried so far?

OT works the best, but is not funded. She has a sensory swing in her room, and the brushing helps.

5. What has been the most difficult part of your child's diagnosis and what would make it easier for you?

I get frustrated with her lack of memory. She forgets where she puts things and often leaves messes everywhere. It is also hard to balance her activity level. How bad is her migraine today? Should I make her do chores or allow her to rest? I have to put the dishwasher on when she is out of the house. I can't clean up when she is home, or it grates on her nervous system like fingernails on a chalkboard. I cannot talk on the phone, it bugs her immensely. If she is asleep any little noise will wake her up. I can't, nor can her brother, sing in the house. He can't play his instrument, it gives his sister a headache. We are always "walking on eggshells".

6. How has your child's diagnosis affected them/yourself socially and emotionally?

She has low self-esteem. She "makes it through the day" at school and falls apart at home. In sheer exhaustion, she will collapse in her bed or on the couch.

7. Has your child's school been supportive or helpful and how? Do you have 504 plan or IEP?

School doesn't see much of her problems even though she HATES school. She is quiet and obedient at school and her problems come out when she gets home. I am currently fighting for her to get an IEP (she has SPD, high anxiety and ADD), but because she is quiet, polite and bright, she gets no help. She is not a discipline problem in the classroom. She has the "freeze", out of the fight, flight or freeze. Often when she is asked if she is ok, Ali will say "yes", but really she is not. She is unable to advocate for herself. She is really good at putting on a mask and making things look fine, when in reality she is in agony.

8. Has there been a positive outcome from your child's diagnosis?

Yes, and no. It is good to finally have acknowledgement that there is an issue, that what she has is real. But there is no help for her.

9. What would you like the general public to know about this situation?

That it is real. That kids that "hold things inside until they finally burst" need help too. That our provincial government provides absolutely no funding.

10. If there is anything else you would like to share with our readers on the subject, not included above, please add it here.

Hayley Kairewich

Chittenango, NY USA

1. When did you first notice your child had Sensory Processing Disorder? When and how was he/she officially diagnosed?

We noticed something was not 100% when she was an infant. She would sleep 20 - 22 hours a day for the first full 2 years of her life but still somehow hitting all childhood milestones like rolling over, sitting up etc. We now know her system was on overload all the time and shutting down by sleeping. Then at 2½ something switched - not sure what, doctors can't tell us that either. She decided to stay up 20 hours out of the day and barely sleep - miserable, crazy meltdowns and tantrums. Everyone told me it's just her terrible two's but deep down I knew it was more. I would constantly ask the doctors and daycare teachers but everyone said she is such a sweetie and always wants to help the adults. So as her family, we got the meltdowns and everyone else got the great behavior! This went on until kindergarten when I couldn't handle the constant issues. She was constantly in and out of the principal's office because of negative behavior. She might have been there 10 times that first year in school and now was almost there on a daily basis. It took a year to get into an OT when she was finally diagnosed at the age of 6 in October of 2012. Within the first five minutes the OT could tell she had severe sensory defensiveness SPD and she was a sensory seeker. The OT put her hand on my knee and asked me how we could go almost 4 years like this and still be sane. At that point I was validated that I wasn't a terrible parent because that was all I heard from everyone all along - "She is great for me, you must be a terrible parent if that is when all of her meltdowns are!"

2. How has this impacted your child's/family's lives?

Well it has impacted our family in a HUGE way. For a long time we were constantly screaming at each other because we were beyond stressed that something wasn't right but no one was listening. Our family would be torn apart because she would have yet another meltdown and we were confined to our house. We couldn't go out in public because it would throw her over the sensory edge and she would throw a temper tantrum/have a meltdown. She would also hate being in the house so no one was ever happy no matter what we were doing. My other two daughters suffered because we couldn't get out, my youngest is terrified of other people/strangers because she was always sheltered inside the house. Now that we know what most of the sensory issues are, for the most part we can avoid some triggers. But still we don't go out to family events - amusement parks, fairs, museums even a pool/lake to swim. They throw her over the edge still. So we have lost a lot of friends because people think we are babying her when in fact it's not worth (for anyone - her or us) sending her into a meltdown. Hopefully we will be able to do some more things - we will get there one day. And hopefully we will find friends that accept us as we are because we aren't changing for anyone!

3. *Do you feel you have a good support system? What could improve a parent's support system?*

No we don't have a support system at all. My husband and I have each other and that's it. None of our family on either side helps or supports us and we have lost many friends. They feel we are babying her and letting her drama win in every situation. We haven't had any time off for a "date" in the past four years. I would love for someone to reach out and say, "I'll take the kids for a few hours or night so you guys can sleep in or go out to dinner and a movie." Or even support along the lines of someone coming over during a meltdown so people see what truly is going on and that I'm not a bad Mom. The stares and negative comments really hurt. Or new strategies for keeping OT fun and new at home. I would love to find another Mom in my community (not in the virtual world - sorry Facebook) that I could call or go over to their house if life is getting crazy with meltdown stress and for someone to say "I understand what you are going through." I would love to have a SPD awareness local chapter where we can help parents and children cope. And not one that is an hour and a half drive to get there. (That is what we have currently- and my daughter hates the car!) I am going to start a support group for all disabilities with our Special Education PTSA I am a member of. We cannot be the only family in this area with SPD. There has to be more either diagnosed or undiagnosed!

4. What has been the best advice and/or treatment you have heard or tried

so far?

Horseback riding has been the best OT for my daughter - she is an animal whisper and has a way with horses! She is like a completely different kid around horses and right after she rides. Her body feels "normal" in her words and not like her skin is crawling. It is very emotional to see the love she has for the horses and how much the horses have love back for her. She has only been riding since November of 2012 and already has enough experience (she is GOOD) and self- confidence/esteem (which she never has!) to enter into a competition. She asked to do it herself - not with any prompting on my end whatsoever.

5. What has been the most difficult part of your child's diagnosis and what

would make it easier for you?

The unknowns of when the meltdowns will come. Even though you try to avert every sensory issue out there (which is exhausting) something that has never been an issue before now triggers her. I wish I could stay one step ahead of her, maybe I will get there one day. The meltdowns tend to happen at the worst possible time also. Maybe more education as to what triggers meltdowns - and ways to try and stop meltdowns before they completely get out of control. More awareness in the community about what SPD is and why kids might be acting the way they do.

6. How has your child's diagnosis affected them/yourself socially

and emotionally?

Yes! My daughter cannot make friends. She has tried but she hasn't been successful. It eats her alive that her older sister can make friends no issues and she can't. She is in social groups but still nothing. I even became her Girl Scout leader (one because I knew no one would be able to handle her and two because I wanted her to have a close group of friends). We have a hard time having people over to our house (play dates for kids or dinners with friends) because she always ends up having a meltdown and friends get scared away. So yes, we have become homebodies that tend to not really go anywhere. And excuses are made when people invite us out.   Even when I explain why we can't they still ask which is disheartening. When we are in public I'm too occupied watching what she is doing and attempting to avoid meltdowns to talk or have a conversation. Even if I get to the comfort level of talking, one of my three daughters will interrupt me and my mind wanders (so many things going on) so I cannot carry a conversation. People tend to not ask us back because of it.

7. *Has your child's school been supportive or helpful and how? Do you have 504 plan or IEP?*

We do have a 504 plan at school where she is getting OT once a week for 30 minutes in a group setting. But the OT that advocated for her is no longer employed by the school district. Now that she is in second grade we feel we may need to advocate/push hard for an IEP because the 504 in New York doesn't hold any grounds legally - it is only followed if the teacher feels like it.   I have been told by the Special Education department that they wouldn't give her an IEP because her diagnosis isn't real because it didn't come from a MD, it came from an OT. This "fighting" advocating for her is long, stressful and exhausting but I will do it as long as it's needed. Second grade is going to be a tough year for her. I saw my now third grader struggle with second grade work last year and she LOVES school. My SPD second grader could care less about school and gets "good grades" but I have a feeling she is going to have issues this year. I want to say she will do great but the work load is intense.

8. *Has there been a positive outcome from your child's diagnosis?*

Yes, we understand her better and when she is starting attitude or a meltdown we understand why now - whereas before we had no clue and thought we were doing something wrong. We can also talk about what triggered her after the meltdown when everyone has calmed down. We also know that communication is key! If you can communicate on a daily basis with the school and with the teacher, life will be a little bit easier. We also go in before school starts to have her see the classroom and meet her teacher. We have her tell the teacher about her diagnosis with her own words then we give her information about it. We tell the teacher what has worked and what hasn't. We are also part of the teacher selection process, giving the principal our daughter's needs/likes and concerns about teachers. That has also helped. Without those in place I feel it would be a lot harder. We only do this now because of her diagnosis - the more education about SPD the better off everyone in the world is.

9. What would you like the general public to know about this situation?

SPD is a real diagnosis that affects the child's brain and it affects not only the child but the whole family. Stares and negative comments are not needed! If anything a helpful hand would be best or just stay away if you can't do that. Support and education is the key to coping with SPD! Without a support system, life is sooooooo hard! So just be there for people who might be learning how to cope with this disorder. Education is important so people grow up being empathetic to people who might be a little different on the inside but don't seem all that different on the outside.

10. If there is anything else you would like to share with our readers on the subject, not included above, please add it here.

Thanks for letting me write about our 7 year old SPD daughter and her life thus far. It is therapeutic for me to put it on paper. It brings up many different emotions that we have been through over the years but I know we are going in the right direction. It is heartwarming to see how far we have come already even though we still have a long way to go.

Poems

Dear Parents of Typical Children:

I know you think your feelings and imagined dramas are more important than my time, but let me explain to you how my days go.

I wake up in the middle of the night to a screaming child. She climbs into bed with me or screams until I go to her. She pushes my spouse out of our bed.

We have no time to ourselves, even in sleep.

In the mornings, I have to follow a strict routine. One deviation causes a meltdown.

I have to make sure all clothes are well worn and all tags have been removed. She cannot wear jeans. She can only wear sweats or leggings. She cannot stand the seams in socks. I often have to turn them inside out. No, I didn't accidentally send my kid to school with inside-out socks. It was on purpose and I thank you to not mention it.

She can't stand having her teeth brushed and often bites the toothbrush or my finger.

I have to give her multiple medications every day. I never thought I would give my child medication, but the alternative was a lot worse. At 5 years old, she swallows pills and has for the last two years. That's better than her spraying my face with the liquid medication she used to be on.

She goes to school and I pray that I won't have a bad report. Some days I am lucky and she only has one incident. The incident usually stems from someone trying to touch her and it going awry.

When she is touched or tugged on by your child, she will retaliate. Yes, my child may seem like an animal to you. I understand her. If you touched me and pulled on me unexpectedly, I wouldn't like it either. But to her, it feels like nails or someone punching her in the face when she is suddenly grabbed.

How would you react to being punched in the face?

I pick her up from school and on a good day, she has wild emotions ranging from sadness to anger to extreme joy. On a bad day, I often have to restrain her. Sometimes for an hour, I have to physically hold her down until she falls asleep.

She has therapies every week and they are increasing in number. She is getting clumsier and they don't know why her muscles are degenerating. She falls and hurts herself every week. I drive her back and forth to the hospital to get these therapies, which cost me thousands of dollars out of pocket every week.

You wondered why I don't have the nice clothes you do or new anything. Now you know.

I can't go to Target, Walmart, Ross or anywhere else with fluorescent lights. As soon as I am in there, she starts yelling, screaming or melting down.

What you may perceive as a temper tantrum is not caused by her being a spoiled child who was told NO when she didn't get her way. It is caused by her being on sensory overload.

I know you probably think that sensory overload is just some excuse. I am here to tell you, it is very real.

Lights, touch, noise, smells. These things are all things typical people are exposed to every day. No one likes a smelly garbage can. That is not THIS.

My child can smell wonderful vanilla cookies baking in the oven and can lose physical control of her body. She can hear the most beautiful song and have to cover her ears and scream.

You can give her a hug because you are happy to see her only to have her start bawling nonstop for an hour.

THIS is what her life is like. This is what MY life is like.

So, excuse me if your current made up gossip and drama in your life does not warrant me taking time out of my day to hear you bitch about why you are unhappy with me.

I apologize if I seem unwilling to allow you to try to walk all over me and throw me under the bus, but the truth is: NOTHING YOU CAN DO TO ME WILL HURT ME.

I have far more important things to handle here.

God. My family.

These are what matter to me.

And, yes, it does hurt me when you don't ask my child to play with yours... even when you've promised many times to do so.

But you know what? It hardly matters.

What matters most is that my child gets all the love, attention and care so that her years on this Earth are the best they can be.

No, I won't allow you to use any of MY time to complain about your problem with me. I simply don't care.

Signed,

A Mother to an Absolutely Awesome Atypical

Written by Laura Limon

These Are Some Things About SPD :

Every morning it starts out rough,
My anxiety is bothering me, I've had enough,
I can't take a bath it hurts too much,
There are just things I cannot touch.

To wear any clothes they're itchy and hard,
I have to be naked, can't play in the yard,
I have no friends I play all alone,
I hope to have more by the time I've grown.

I never sit still anymore at school,
No way to focus without a sensory tool,
Acting bad in class to hide my shame,
I can't hold a pencil or spell my name.

Lights for me are just too bright,
Makes me panic and hold mom tight,
Many sounds really bother me,
I have spd can't you all see.

There are many things I have to avoid,
Some were things that I once enjoyed,
I don't want hugs and I will wipe off your kiss,
being affectionate I sometimes miss.

I don't like the way that some things smell,
I don't speak so I cannot tell,
I overreact to cuts and bug bites,
I am still a child, I do have rights.

Many think I can control how I feel,
They don't believe spd is real,
I always feel the need to chew,
I bite on everything that's what I do.

I avoid using my hands for messy play,
I wish these sensations would just go away,
With my food I am very picky,
I don't like food that's salty or sticky.

I avoid brushing my teeth and my hair,
Some of these things are so unfair,
It's sometimes tough buttoning and zipping my clothes, I can't put up
my hair or use hair bows.

Sometimes I get embarrassed and I blush,
This will get better if I use my brush,
Brushing every two hours every single day,
My OT says it will all get better this way.
`
Jumping, bouncing, I like to climb,
This will all get better in time,
I am so hyper I can't sit still,
For me to be calm I take a pill.

I make some noises I love to stim,
My hair and nails I don't want to trim,
These are some things about spd,
They make me special, they make me, me.

Written By Jeanette Baker

We'd like to give thanks to God who gives us strength. A huge thank you to our cover designer, Christina Fuselli, and our editor, Jayne Reynolds. You both are amazing! To our beautiful children, Bean, Gavin, Emilio and Emmett, you all are true heroes who, despite your challenges, continue to soar; you all are precious blessings we love so much and thank God for every day! To our families and friends, your encouragement, love and support is what made these pages possible. And a special thank you to all the parents and caregivers who contributed a survey, your stories are inspirations to us all.

Links and More:

Upcoming books in the Questions from those who Know series:
-Autism
-Oppositional Defiant Order
-ADHD/ADD
*And More

If you or someone you know would like to be featured in an upcoming book.
Please visit: surveyforbooks.com

Facebook Links:

Questions from those who Know Facebook page:

https://www.facebook.com/pages/QUESTIONS-from-those-who-KNOW-Cindy-Jusino-Jeanette-Baker/691434924214610

Sensory Processing Disorder Parent Support Facebook page:
https://www.facebook.com/sensoryprocessingdisorderparentsupport

Cindy Jusino's Facebook author page:
https://www.facebook.com/CindyJusinoAuthor

Website Links:

Questions from those who Know official webpage:
QuestionsfromthosewhoKnow.com

Jeanette's website for everything related to SPD:
http://sensoryprocessing.yolasite.com/

Cindy's author website:
http://www.cindyjusino.com

Other books by Cindy Jusino:

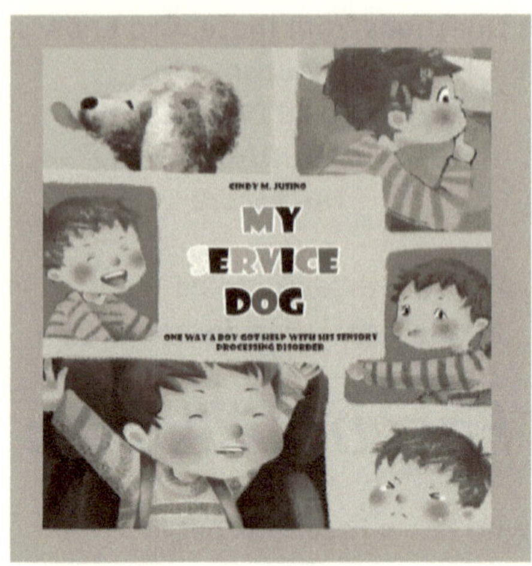

My Service Dog: Help for Sensory Processing Disorder.

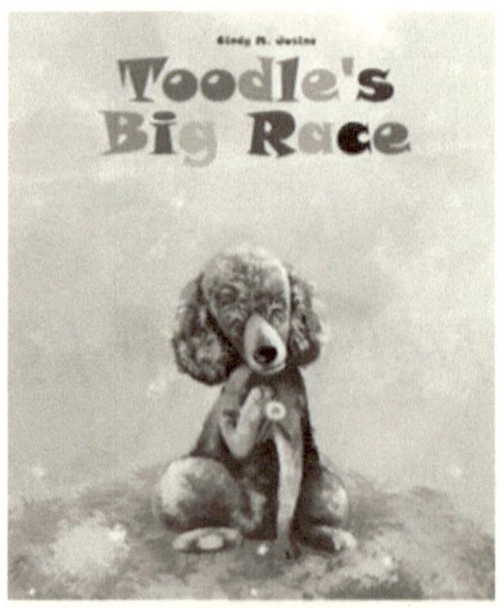

Toodles Big Race: Interactive for children that don't like to sit still!

Available on BarnesandNoble.com